THE LEADERSHIP PRESCRIPTION

HOW HIGH-PERFORMING CLINICIANS BECOME VISIONARY LEADERS

Maia D. Carter,
MD, MPH, FACP, FACHE

The Leadership Prescription:
How High-Performing Clinicians Become Visionary Leaders

Written by Maia D. Carter, MD, MPH, FACP, FACHE

Design and cover art by Peaceful Profits.

Paperback ISBN: 979-8-9948445-0-2
eBook ISBN: 979-8-9948445-1-9
Hardcover ISBN: 979-8-9948445-2-6

Advanced Praise for *The Leadership Prescription: How High-Performing Clinicians Become Visionary Leaders*

The Leadership Prescription: How High-Performing Clinicians Become Visionary Leaders is the mentor, the playbook, and the push you've been waiting for. With practical frameworks, authentic storytelling, and a refreshing dose of courage, Dr. Maia Carter offers clinicians a clear and compassionate path into leadership. Her voice is both empowering and actionable. She reminds us that leadership isn't about perfection, but about persistence and vision. This book is a must-read for every clinician ready to step confidently into their next chapter.

–Dr. Kimberly Foxworth, DNP, EMHA, MSN, CCRN, RCIS, CPHQ, NEA-BC, FACHE Saint Lukes Hospital Chief Nursing & Quality Executive

Clinician leadership makes all the difference in healthcare. This book is a clear, practical guide that helps clinicians move past the fear of change and step confidently into leadership, while reminding us that growth can be done with grace, confidence, and even in cute, comfortable shoes!

–Andrea Davis, CEO, Viticus Group

In this remarkable work, Dr. Maia Carter distills the wisdom, discipline, and compassion that have defined her distinguished career as both a clinician and healthcare executive. Having personally benefited from her coaching, I found her insights both transformative and profoundly practical. As I read on, I recognized my own journey—from the challenges of full-time clinical practice to the many roles I have thrived in as a physician leader—and I felt seen. This book offers an essential road map for physicians aspiring to leadership positions, as well as for those seeking to strengthen their impact through private practice. Dr. Carter has created an inspiring and highly actionable guide that empowers physicians to lead with the purpose, balance, and vision critically needed in today's complex healthcare landscape.

–Luis H. Medina-Garcia, MD, FIDSA
Founder, Academic Infectious Disease Physicians; Founding President, Southern Nevada Infectious Disease Society; Program Director, Infectious Diseases Fellowship; Southern Hills Hospital

This is a compelling guide for those perplexed about building confidence and for many practical steps forward into healthcare leadership. It is a great fit for clinicians of any age moving from contemplation to preparation to action, in stages of career change. I wish I had had this book to absorb when I first made the change from full time clinical work to a salaried medical director role. The coaching option Dr. Carter presents would have accelerated my career faster, enabling me to be more ready when my next promotion came.

–Prentiss Taylor, MD, FACP
Chief Medical Editor, Oakstone Continuing Medical Education Program, Attending Physician at Advocate Health Care; Former Regional Medical Director

DEDICATION

To every clinician who felt the call to lead not because it was easy, but because it was necessary.

Not because you had it all figured out, but because something inside you knew you were meant for more.

This book is for the ones who dared to step beyond their comfort zones.

For those who stayed after rounds to ask the harder questions, who challenged the status quo not to be disruptive, but to make things better, who learned to lead not just with protocols and precision, but with empathy, courage, and conviction.

It's for the clinician who wrestled with imposter syndrome, who led anyway. For the ones who sat in meetings and thought,

"There has to be a better way" and decided to be part of creating it.

You chose purpose over position. Vision over comfort.

And progress over perfection.

May you continue to rise with integrity,

lead with clarity, and never forget that your clinical roots, your time at the bedside, the lives you've touched, and the teams you've served are not left behind. They are the very foundation of your strategic brilliance.

In addition, this book is for any high-performing professional who's ever wondered: *What's next for me and do I have what it takes to lead at the next level?* Whether you're a clinician, educator, entrepreneur, or executive, this is your invitation to rise into strategic leadership with clarity and courage.

To my coaches, mentors, mentees, friends, and family, thank you.

Your wisdom, belief, and unwavering support helped shape every word in these pages. I am deeply grateful for your presence on this journey.

With Gratitude,
Maia D. Carter, MD, MPH, FACP, FACHE

FOREWORD

By Erica Scavella, MD, FACP, FACHE
Senior Executive Physician Leader

Carpe diem—seize the day. This Latin phrase has guided my life, not as a cliché but as a compass.

This book, authored by my colleague Dr. Maia Carter, is not just a reflection of her path. It is a guide for yours. Dr. Carter has walked the road from frontline physician to strategic leader. She knows what it means to feel the tension between clinical identity and the pull of leadership. She has lived the challenges, faced the doubts, and emerged with wisdom that is both practical and profound. Authenticity, clarity, and resilience are the very truths that echo throughout *The Leadership Prescription.*

What makes this work extraordinary is not only her expertise but her authenticity. She does not offer leadership as a lofty ideal. She offers it as a lived truth—grounded in stories, frameworks, and tools that will empower you to step into leadership with courage and confidence.

This book is both a mirror and a road map: It reflects the struggles many clinicians face in their leadership journey while guiding them toward new ways of thinking, leading, and thriving.

As you turn these pages, prepare to be challenged. Prepare to see yourself differently. And most importantly, prepare to seize your own day.

The wisdom Dr. Carter shares is not meant to be read passively. It is meant to be lived. If you lean into these lessons with openness and courage, you will discover that the power to lead was always within you.

So to every reader: Seize your day. Lead with clarity. Show up as your whole, authentic self. The world is waiting, and it needs nothing less than the leader only you can be.

"If your actions inspire others to dream more, learn more, do more and become more, then you are a leader."

–John Quincy Adams, 6th President of the United States

TABLE OF CONTENTS

INTRODUCTION

Envisioning the Leader Within

This book exists to help high-performing clinicians envision the leader in themselves. I had to learn how to envision myself as a leader before I could become a leader, someone who is a confident, influential change agent.

There I was in my habitual rhythm, seeing patients back-to-back and enjoying it. After all, seeing the patients was the fun part; the administrative burden that accompanied it was nauseating and heralded the real risk of burnout. The administrators regarded me as someone who could easily create rapport with the patients. I was the kind of physician who came in early and stayed late. I stayed focused and prided myself on clinical excellence.

That rhythm felt safe and familiar, like a well-worn pair of scrubs. But beneath the surface, I sensed a pull toward something more—a chance to shape healthcare beyond the exam room. Maybe you're feeling that pull too. You're exceptional at patient care, trusted by your patients and colleagues, yet you wonder if there's a bigger role for you, one where your ideas can transform systems, teams, and lives. This book is for you—the clinician who's ready to step into leadership but hesitates, unsure if you have what it takes.

I'm here to tell you: You do. I'm living proof, and by the end of this journey, you'll see the proof in yourself.

One day, I was diligently taking care of one of my patients when my supervisor came in, asked me politely to step out of the exam room, and told me about a new leadership role. This opportunity was open for all who met the minimal criteria to apply, and he shared it not only with me but also each of my peers. He went on to say that this position would be responsible for recruitment and retention of clinicians, shoring up preventative health measures, partnering with other disciplines, and ensuring timely access to patient care. Immediately, I got excited and thought that this would be a great opportunity for me to finally share my ideas and make the changes that I had been wanting to see in our clinics for quite some time.

Suddenly, my heart started to race, and I thought to myself that I didn't have any formal management training. I was a single mom juggling two toddlers, and I wasn't sure I had it in me to lead my physician peers. I thought about the data and strongly doubted my ability to decipher complex data on graphs in order to create impact. And then, the thought of having to lay down the law over a bunch of physicians sounded like a headache to me. Overwhelmed by the obstacles I saw, I politely told my supervisor that I was flattered, but that type of role was just not for me. I swiftly went back into my exam room and resumed care with my patient.

That moment was a crossroads. The excitement I felt was real, but so was the fear. It's the same fear you might be facing—fear of stepping into the unknown, of failing, of not being "enough."

But here's the truth: That fear is a sign you're on the edge of something transformative. Let me share a story to bring this home. Dr. Sarah, an ob-gyn, was offered a chance to lead her hospital's women's health program. Like me, she was thrilled but paralyzed by doubt. "I'm great with patients, but I've never led a team," she expressed. She worried about managing budgets and navigating politics. Through coaching, she learned to reframe her fear as a signal of growth. She applied, leaned on her clinical expertise, and won the role, thus proving that leadership isn't about having all the answers—it's about trusting your ability to find them.

When I was approached about the leadership role, I was flattered—but also uncertain. I would be competing against other more experienced physicians who had both management training and experience under their belt. I went home and discussed it with my personal board of directors, my parents. After my divorce, my parents were the only two people in the world that I trusted. This local organization had not seen a leader that looked like me or sounded like me, and they definitely hadn't had a woman leader who was divorced with two babies. The board deliberated, and the decision was to apply for the position. With the board having my back, I mustered up enough confidence to garner a shift in my mindset.

That support was everything. It reminded me I wasn't alone, and you aren't either. Your "board of directors"—whether family, friends, or mentors—can help you see the leader you're becoming.

Try this tool to tap into that support: **The Confidence Council Exercise**. Identify three people in your life who believe in your potential. Schedule a conversation with each and ask, "What strengths do you see in me that would make me a great leader?" Write down their answers and revisit them when doubt creeps in. This council will anchor you, just as my parents did, giving you the courage to shift your mindset.

I dwelled on the idea of how great it would be to sit in the driver's seat. The thought of managing operations and creating an environment for patients and staff that was mutually beneficial was inspirational. The thought of optimizing customer service, working toward optimal collaboration between physicians and other disciplines was exciting to me. Hiring clinicians that were the best fit for the organization sounded empowering. Creating a smooth experience for new physicians coming into the organization was appealing. It would be great to build relationships with other managers so we could work better together and actually make progress. I began to envision myself in the driver's seat, making positive moves for the organization.

That vision was the spark. It's the same spark you need to ignite your leadership journey. Imagine yourself leading a team, presenting a bold idea, or shaping policies that improve patient care. That vision isn't a fantasy—it's a preview of your future. To make it real, try **The Vision Spark Meditation**. Find a quiet moment, close your eyes, and picture yourself as a confident clinician-leader. Where are you? What are you doing? How do you feel? Write down three words that describe this version of you—perhaps "bold," "impactful," or "authentic." Keep these words where you'll see them daily, like your phone or desk, to fuel your transformation.

THE INTERVIEW

As I prepared for the interview, a friend of mine challenged me and asked me why I wanted this job. After all, the reality is that most folks do not want this type of role with so much responsibility. That triggered me to dig deep and answer that for myself. I realized later that the answer to that question was critical during my interview to clearly convey my motivations.

The interview room had a serious, intense energy. There were five men and one woman, all seasoned top managers. My heart was racing, and I began to feel sweat under my arms. I did my best to answer each question and leveraged personal insights I had from working in the clinic and tools I developed informally to help streamline care. The questions I so dutifully prepared to answer were not the questions presented. The interview shifted to the topic I dreaded the most: data. They asked me how much I knew about data. Data was not something that was taught or expected during my medical training. I stated that I had limited knowledge of the databases that were used in the organization. However, I knew how important it was to monitor success in caring for patients. I was so glad when that interview was over. I sat in my car for 20 minutes critically reviewing every question that was asked and my corresponding answer.

That interview was a crucible, testing my resilience. You'll face similar moments—interviews, presentations, or tough conversations—that push you to your edge. But those moments don't define your worth; they reveal your growth. Dr. Sarah, from earlier, faced a grueling interview for her leadership role. She stumbled on a question about financial metrics but recovered by tying it to her passion for patient outcomes. Her authenticity won the panel over. You can do the same by preparing not for perfection but for presence. Try the **Interview Power Prep**. Before any high-stakes moment, write down three key strengths (e.g., empathy, problem-solving) and one personal story that showcases each. Practice sharing these aloud to build confidence and authenticity.

GETTING THE JOB

In spite of my own self-doubts, after all the scores were counted, I got the job. I instantly started shaking with both excitement and anxiety, because from that point on, I knew the trajectory of my career would be forever changed. I would not be that girl who could quietly see patients and mind her business. My colleagues were suddenly my subordinates. These were just some of the challenges that I would be facing on this new leadership journey.

CHAPTER 1

From Clinical Comfort to Leadership Courage

The beginning of my leadership journey was full of anxiety, especially since at my core, I am an introvert. I never knew what I was going to be faced with each week. There would be conduct or performance issues I needed to address. There were key messages that I needed to send to our executive leadership team. Everything moved so fast. Mostly, I was nervous about getting caught off guard, being asked a question that I was not prepared for.

I was used to excelling at my clinical expertise, my comfort zone. I had to be patient with myself as I began to acquire more strategic expertise. I remember looking over at my clinical staff thinking, *Boy, that clinical work seems easy peasy compared to these leadership duties I am doing now.* Although I was humbled to have the role, I quickly learned that I was in a sink or swim environment.

There was no clear road map on how I, as a clinician, could be successful in leadership. I recall many times walking back to my office after attending an important meeting with my head down, discouraged. I needed the next experience to be better. So, I reviewed the meeting with my administrative staff and slowly put together the pieces and players of the organization. That's where I made the decision that I was going to swim.

As the first year progressed, I started to become more transparent about what I did not understand, including the leadership vocabulary, like the difference between strategic initiative and tactical initiative or how to best use the terms manpower and resource request.One of my gifts was my likability or my ability to connect with people easily. There always seemed to be someone who was willing to take the time to explain terms, organizational roles, and organizational priorities and challenges. All I needed to do was muster up the courage to ask.

One day, I was in the nurse executive's office, and I saw a journal on her desk. It was the *Journal of Healthcare Management* from the American College of Healthcare Executives. It was composed of articles that spoke directly about the types of issues I was addressing at work, like change management and leading people.

My heart fluttered, and I knew I needed this journal in my life. That day, I joined the American College of Healthcare Executives. This organization became one of the major tools for my growth in leadership strategy and principles. If you recall, I made the decision that I was going to swim. By empowering myself with resources and a solid network, I began to float, then one stroke at a time, coming up for air, with the sea (empowering resources and network) holding me up, I began to swim.

Two years into the journey, I would get the kids off to school and walk confidently into the office. I remember one particular outfit was a nicely fitted purple suit that laid over my body shape well. I felt comfortable and commanded respect. I had heels that were cute but also comfortable. I promised myself I would never buy any shoes that did not pass the "cc" test—cute *and* comfortable. My colleagues would tease me and tell me that they knew I was in the building before they actually saw me, because they heard my heels against the hallway floors. I walked with a smile, even when feeling anxious.

Year by year in my leadership journey, I created a habit of intentionally giving myself positive self-talk and uttering an affirmation under my breath: "You can do it," or "You got this." During morning leadership huddles, I spoke confidently about the current state of clinic operations, staffing, and anything else I needed to bring to executive leadership. I was often tossed an impromptu or unexpected question. This was very uncomfortable for me, since I like to be prepared and know what to expect. Each time, I answered to the best of my ability. After being thrown a few curveballs, it finally became routine for me to be compassionate and less critical of myself as I got more comfortable answering questions off the top of my head.

This self-compassion did not come automatically. It grew over time and was very intentional. I would say to myself, "Girl, you are okay. You answered the question to the best of your ability. You were confident and honest. Mission accomplished. Now you have a little more information about what types of things you may need to convey. It will be even better next time." Also, as I grew a good reputation of integrity amongst my leadership peers, I had seasoned allies at the table who often spoke up and supported me in addressing the curveball. Self-compassion became easier once I realized that I was not alone.

I learned how to have strategic relationships with my colleagues. That involved knowing the roles key members played in the organization and how their roles impacted my goals and, ultimately, the care of our patients. Finding common priorities and building on ideas was key.

It was important for me to listen more than I spoke, so I could understand perspectives and competing priorities amongst different disciplines and programs. I valued the team who reported to me and counted on their feedback as I developed strategy. They counted on me to help develop professional growth and to delegate tasks to them. Things started to feel better when I focused on a growth mindset and forwent the perfection mindset. Leadership was a marathon and not a race. I started to get excited about getting stronger due to what I learned each day. As the years progressed and I started to refine my craft, I found that other rising leaders came to me for advice and guidance. I slowly began a shift toward sharing my acquired knowledge with others and, ultimately, becoming a coach.

THE MINDSET SHIFT: FROM CLINICIAN TO STRATEGIC THINKER

Let me pause here to share a critical insight that transformed my journey and will be the cornerstone of your success as a clinician leader: You must shift from a practitioner mindset to a strategic thinker mindset.

As clinicians, we're trained to focus on precision, mastery, and immediate patient outcomes. We thrive in controlled environments where our expertise is our shield. But leadership? It's a different beast. It's about embracing ambiguity, thinking beyond the exam room, and aligning your actions with the bigger picture—whether that's organizational goals, patient population health, or systemic change.

This mindset shift doesn't happen overnight. For me, it started with small, intentional steps. I began asking myself, "What's the broader impact of my decisions? How do my actions today shape the future of my team, my organization, or my patients?" These questions forced me to step out of my clinical comfort zone and into a space where I had to think like a chess player, anticipating moves three steps ahead.

If you're reading this and feeling overwhelmed by the leap from clinical excellence to leadership, know this: *You already have the skills to succeed*. Your ability to diagnose, problem-solve, and connect with people as a clinician is the foundation. The key is redirecting those skills toward strategic goals.

CASE STUDY: PAM

My colleague Pam was already in leadership when I met her. She was strong, and she had a captivating presence and a heart of gold. But she wanted a change. Pam was miserable in her current position but stayed, because it was more comfortable than leaving that role and taking a risk into unknown territory.

She dreaded getting up and going to work every day just to be consumed with guilt. Pam knew that the job no longer inspired her, and it left many of her true talents untapped. At the same time, it took precious time away from her children.

Over time, this dead-end job bled into precious time she needed for her family. Time with her family was a big priority for her. She wanted more of a challenge career-wise, yet she had key nonnegotiable family obligations that came into play. I definitely could relate to her, as my children have always been at the forefront of my decision-making. Through my signature methodology, I was able to help her uncover an opportunity that fit right into her untapped talents, provided her with economic impact, and allowed her time with family. I created a customized road map to help her land her new position. If you are in a role that is no longer interesting or is unaligned with your gifts, just like Pam, I can help you too.

Actionable Takeaway for You: If you're feeling stuck like Pam, start by identifying one talent or passion that's lying dormant in your current role. Write it down. Then, ask yourself: *What's one small step I can take this week to align my work with this talent?* It could be as simple as scheduling a coffee chat with a colleague in a department that excites you or researching a leadership course that sparks your interest. Small steps lead to big shifts.

CASE STUDY: DELORES

Another colleague, Delores, was desperately suffering from burnout. Her work environment sucked. Her peers had bad attitudes and called off repeatedly, leaving her to do both her job and theirs. This was coupled with frustrations of being in a system that had a huge resource deficit, which impaired her ability to support her patients like she wanted. We spent a fair amount of time creating a clear career vision, exploring skills, and identifying personal priorities. Don't worry, I will tell you all about this in chapters 6 and 8. She entered a training program that would launch her into a position that would rejuvenate her, not deplete her. As a clinical leader, she trusted her leadership identity and boldly took those next steps to make a career move that honored her values, health, and well-being.

Actionable Takeaway for You: Burnout is a signal, not a sentence. Like Delores, take ten minutes today to write down your non-negotiables—your health, your values, your vision for your career. Then, identify one resource (a course, a mentor, a professional organization) that can help you move toward a role that aligns with those priorities. You deserve a career that energizes you, not one that drains you.

CASE STUDY: JASON

Jason discussed with me his desire to excel and go up the chain but was stuck in a taskmaster mindset. This taskmaster mindset hindered him from emerging into his true identity as a leader. His leadership position required him to delegate many of these tasks to his subordinates. However, he found himself getting overwhelmed, offering his help, overextending himself, and getting burned out. Being overbusy with multiple tasks left him unable to prioritize the things that would help him emerge as a leader.

I shared with him my **Leadership Arsenal** and helped him understand that in order to emerge into the thought leader he wanted to become, he needed to free himself of being the ultimate taskmaster and learn new skills that would challenge him and garner his growth. I discuss more about this **Leadership Arsenal** in chapter 4. Through my coaching, he realized that a negative outcome of the taskmaster mindset would be stealing opportunity from others in both accomplishing work and building confidence. He realized he needed to revamp a success circle around him to build community and hold him accountable. Don't worry, I will get more into being free of the taskmaster mindset and having great people in place in chapters 4 and 6.

Actionable Takeaway for You: If you're caught in a taskmaster trap like Jason, try this: Delegate one small task this week that someone else on your team can handle. Use the time you free up to focus on a strategic goal—perhaps drafting a proposal for a new initiative or preparing for a high-level meeting. Delegation isn't just about offloading work; it's about empowering others and elevating yourself.

BUILDING YOUR LEADERSHIP FOUNDATION

I help clinicians like you reach your leadership goals, because I completely understand many of the challenges, both intrinsic and extrinsic, that you are going through. I have been in your shoes. When I trusted my identity as a leader, I began to create my own road map. Although stumbling along the way, and at times feeling like I took five steps back, I kept going. I was willing to swallow the large pill of feedback from mentors, glean information from key organizations, and leverage my network. I slowly started to piece together the building blocks of how not only to present myself as a respected physician but also as a respected organizational leader.

That led me to develop **Dr. Maia Leadership Coaching** that now helps you, my beloved clinician. Oh, what a great feeling it was to create wins for the clinicians I was supervising. I could address and fix many of their frustrations. I activated my gift of connecting with others quickly and finding viable solutions. That was satisfying.

As I matured in my leadership skills, I learned how to speak with authority and in a manner that resonated with my audience. Trust me, my first round of formal presentations was a flop. The naysayers sure had a lot to say those days. However, I had to turn my inner critic into an inner advocate, forcing me to focus on the get-up. Trust me, I learned how to perfect a bounce back, wipe away my tears, and reexamine how to get better at this leadership role.

My confidence grew, and I began to receive affirmation from many other leaders in the organization. The voices of the naysayers got softer and became less significant. Wow, did that feel great. To top it off, I was now earning enough money that allowed me to have choices about where I sent my kids to school. Turns out, moving through fear and uncertainty while resisting the urge to throw in the towel was totally worth it.

YOUR TURN: START SWIMMING

If you're an aspiring clinician leader reading this, you might be feeling the same anxiety I felt, wondering if you're cut out for leadership, afraid of being caught off guard, or unsure how to bridge the gap between clinical expertise and strategic excellence. Here's the truth: *You are proof.* You are proof that the skills you've honed as a clinician, such as empathy, problem-solving, and resilience, can be transformed into leadership superpowers. The secret is in the mindset shift. Start small. Ask one question this week that scares you. Join one professional organization that aligns with your goals. Say one affirmation to yourself before a big meeting. These small actions are the strokes that will help you swim.

In the chapters ahead, I'll share my signature methodology—the **Dr. Maia Leadership Framework**—that will guide you step-by-step from clinical excellence to strategic excellence. You'll learn how to build your **Leadership Arsenal**, create strategic relationships, and trust your leadership identity, just as I did. You'll hear more stories of clinicians like Pam, Delores, and Jason, who transformed their careers and lives by embracing this mindset shift. Most importantly, you'll discover that leadership isn't about being perfect—it's about being persistent, compassionate, and strategic.

Your First Step: Before you move on to the next chapter, take a moment to reflect. Write down one fear that's holding you back from stepping into leadership. Then, write one small action you can take this week to face that fear. Maybe it's reaching out to a mentor, reading an article on strategic leadership, or simply saying "I am proof" in the mirror. Whatever it is, commit to it. You're not just a clinician—you're a leader in the making.

CHAPTER 2

Getting Real With Your Leadership Potential

Upon completing my physician training program, I felt a sense of pride and privilege at the end of the day. I played a valuable role in another person's health. As years progressed in my clinical medicine career, that joy slowly started to fall away. Coming in early and staying late was par for the course, but it got old. I was flooded with charting and the administrative work that comes along with patient care, and this was not discussed in medical school. I needed a change from this environment.

I understood exactly how Pam felt, because I had experienced the exact same feelings during my years as a frontline clinician. I found myself in a job that was no longer fulfilling, and I knew there were other parts of my talent that needed to be tapped. I became frustrated and isolated. However, the mere thought of taking something new was overwhelming. I would be so excited when I saw my clinician colleagues take the step up and into a leadership role. However, it wasn't long until I got disappointed all over again when the status quo failed to change. I was frustrated yet again. I thought to myself: *If I were to get the opportunity to lead, I would do things differently.* I would take additional steps to ensure the systems would work well on a clinician's first day of work. I wanted to help reduce the administrative workload. When I got the opportunity, I knew what I needed to do to ensure that positive changes actually happened once I was in charge. I made those changes for both clinicians and patients, and I am ready to help you do the same.

Have you ever thought about the changes you could impact if you were in charge?

Are you ready to get real with your current reality? Society can get you thinking that since you're a high-functioning clinician, you have reached the pinnacle of success and financial stability, and there is absolutely no reason for you to complain about anything. You are feeling alone and isolated and wear a mask that everything is okay. Perseverance is what is expected of us and what we have been praised for.

I reminisce often with my physician colleagues about how many of us were expected to suppress our feelings and do whatever it took to fulfill the mission, whether it was taking care of a patient or making the grade. On the outside, we look amazing and well put together, but on the inside, we often feel sorrowful, weary, and exhausted. We take in others' expectations of how we should feel; we wear a mask and ignore our true emotions. We have been conditioned through our medical training to satisfy expectations of others at the expense of our own needs. The time is now to acknowledge our own current condition and do something about it.

Over time, the shadow of burnout and lack of autonomy, coupled with ideas of how, if in a leadership role, I could be in the driver's seat to make positive changes, left me envisioning a different role for myself. But quickly, my imposter syndrome got in the way. With no formal management training and experience, a visible leadership role would create a humiliating situation if I made a mistake. There were other clinicians who had MBAs and experience that would be more suited for leadership. With a little help from two people I trusted to remind me of how far I had come and that my ideas were sound, I took the leap to pursue leadership.

Moving into leadership was one of the best decisions of my life for both my career and my family. Initially, achieving the leadership role was a very daunting, emotional, nervous rollercoaster. I learned as I went, often failing to have impact when giving presentations. Oftentimes, I did not understand the management language that happened in meetings. I wasn't able to anticipate what was coming next in the fiscal year and what I was expected to do, and it was nerve-racking. I made mistakes at first, hired folks I should not have, and did not speak up as much as I should have, likely due to imposter syndrome, as seemingly in every space, folks were so much more advanced than I was in the leadership world. However, with each task, I got up, dusted myself off, reflected on my performance and found a way to do it better next time. I learned how to be successful in accomplishing the work of hiring doctors, managing policies, giving presentations, and negotiating work, and the list goes on.

Over time, I welcomed flexibility and the versatility of tasks done as a leader. I am here to be your leadership coach. I am here to help you accomplish the same thing I did. I learned that I didn't need yet another degree before I could move into leadership. I learned how to navigate the leadership waters, and I have charted a course that you can follow too. It's time to get real honest with yourself about your current reality, reveal common pitfalls, and celebrate your accomplishments so that you can streamline your leadership journey.

THE WEIGHT OF THE MASK

Let's talk about that mask we wear as clinicians. You know the one—the polished, professional exterior that screams "I've got it all together" while inside, you're grappling with exhaustion, self-doubt, and the nagging feeling that you're meant for more. I wore that mask for years. I'd walk into the hospital with my crisp white coat, my stethoscope draped just so, and a smile that hid the fact that I was frustrated spending my evenings finishing up notes and spending precious vacation time keeping up with patient test results. I was upset and feeling torn between heading out to the beach with the kids and ensuring I did not miss any critical patient alerts. That realization hit me like a ton of bricks. My family and my well-being were at risk.

If you're nodding along, feeling that same weight, know this: *You are not alone.* The mask is heavy, but it's not permanent. The first step to shedding it is getting honest with yourself. Ask: *What's draining me? What's lighting me up? What do I want my career to look like five years from now?* These questions are scary because they force you to confront the gap between where you are and where you want to be. But they're also liberating. They're the spark that ignites your journey from clinician to leader.

THE MINDSET SHIFT: FROM DOING TO LEADING

Here's where the secret key comes in: It's the mindset shift from practitioner to strategic thinker. As clinicians, we're trained to focus on the task at hand—diagnosing, treating, and documenting. We're doers, and we're darn good at it. But leadership requires a different lens. It's about seeing the big picture, anticipating challenges, and inspiring others to achieve a shared vision. It's about moving from "How do I get this done?" to "How do I empower my team to get this done?"

For me, this shift started with a moment of clarity. I was sitting in a staff meeting, listening to yet another discussion about budget limitations and staffing shortages. I realized that if I stayed in my clinical role, I'd keep complaining about the system without ever changing it.

But as a leader, I could help the system—streamline processes, advocate for my team, and improve patient care from the top down. That realization was my turning point. It wasn't about abandoning my clinical roots; it was about leveraging them to create broader impact.

Actionable Takeaway for You: Take ten minutes this week to write down one change you'd make if you were in charge. Maybe it's reducing administrative burdens, improving staff morale, or implementing a new patient care protocol. Don't censor yourself—dream big. This exercise will help you start thinking like a strategic leader, even before you step into a formal role.

OVERCOMING IMPOSTER SYNDROME

Let's talk about that pesky imposter syndrome. For me, it was a constant whisper: *You're not qualified. You don't have an MBA. You'll mess this up.* I remember my first leadership meeting where I was surrounded by executives tossing around terms like ROI and strategic alignment. I felt like a kid who'd sneakily joined the grown-ups' table. But here's what I learned: *Imposter syndrome is a liar.* Your clinical expertise, your ability to connect with people, your resilience under pressure—**these are leadership qualities.** You don't need a fancy degree to lead; you need courage, curiosity, and a willingness to learn.

I leaned on two trusted colleagues who became my cheerleaders. One was a seasoned administrator who'd seen it all. She'd pull me aside after a meeting and say, "You did fine. Next time, try this." The other was a fellow clinician-turned-leader who reminded me that our patient-centered perspective was our superpower. Their encouragement gave me the confidence to keep going, even when I stumbled.

Actionable Takeaway for You: Identify one person in your network who can be your leadership cheerleader—someone who believes in you and can offer honest feedback. Schedule a coffee chat or a quick call with them this week. Share your leadership aspirations and ask for one piece of advice. That conversation could be the push you need to take your first step.

CASE STUDY: DR. MADISON'S LEAP

Let me share a story about Dr. Madison, a client who reminds me so much of where I started. Dr. Madison was a brilliant Internal Medicine physician who practiced medicine for decades. She dreamed of leading a department but was paralyzed by not being heard by her local leaders and peers. "They are not listening," she'd say. "I don't know why this is not working." Through my coaching, we worked on reframing her mindset. We identified her strengths—her ability to come up with fresh ideas, her knack for simplifying complex problems—and mapped them to effective communication and emotional intelligence leadership skills. Within six months, she was getting the needs of her clinics met successfully. Today, she's thriving, and her team is too.

Actionable Takeaway for You: Like Dr. Madison, make a list of three skills you excel at as a clinician (e.g., problem-solving, empathy, attention to detail). Then, write down how each skill could translate to leadership (e.g., problem-solving becomes strategic planning, empathy becomes team motivation). This exercise will help you see that you're already equipped to lead.

YOUR LEADERSHIP ROAD MAP STARTS HERE

I'm here to tell you that you don't need another degree or a decade of experience to step into leadership. What you need is a road map—and that's exactly what I'm sharing in this book. My **Dr. Maia Leadership Framework** will guide you through the steps I took to move from burnout to breakthrough, from clinician to strategic leader. It's not about being perfect; it's about being persistent. Every mistake I made—every flopped presentation, every misinterpreted management term—was a lesson that made me stronger. And every lesson brought me closer to the leader I am today.

Years into my leadership journey, I stood in my office one day, and I looked at a photo of my kids on my desk. I realized that taking the leap into leadership didn't just transform my career—it gave me the financial freedom to choose the best schools for them and the flexibility to be present for their milestones. It gave me the power to shape a healthcare system to work better for my colleagues and our patients.

Most importantly, it gave me the confidence to know that clinicians like you can become strategic leaders who can change the game.

Your First Step: Before you turn the page, grab a notebook or your phone and answer this question: *What's one thing I'm ready to change about my current reality?* Maybe it's the way you feel at the end of a shift, the lack of influence you have over decisions, or the nagging sense that you're meant for more. Write it down, then add one small action you can take this week to move toward that change—whether it's researching a leadership course, reaching out to a mentor, or simply saying "I am proof" to yourself. That small step is the beginning of your leadership journey.

In the chapters ahead, we'll dive deeper into the **Dr. Maia Leadership Framework**, exploring how to build your **Leadership Arsenal**, navigate imposter syndrome, and create strategic relationships that amplify your impact. You'll hear more stories of clinicians who've walked this path and come out stronger. Most importantly, you'll discover that leadership isn't about having all the answers—it's about asking the right questions and trusting your ability to find the way.

CHAPTER 3

Hurdles—Turning Obstacles into Opportunities

By this time, you are probably thinking about how you would be ecstatic about the influence and decision-making power of making positive changes. However, on the other hand, you are consumed with several perceived hurdles that allow you to be stuck with the feelings of not being able to have success at all. Let's jump in and talk through some of those common hurdles and how, in spite of the challenge, you still can be successful.

THE POWER OF REFRAMING HURDLES

Before we dive into specific hurdles, let's talk about what hurdles really are. As clinicians, we're trained to see obstacles as problems to solve—whether it's a tricky diagnosis or a patient's complex needs. Leadership hurdles are no different. They're not walls; they're stepping stones. Each one is an opportunity to grow, to refine your skills, and to prove to yourself that you're capable of more than you think. My **Dr. Maia Leadership Framework**, which we'll explore throughout this book, is designed to help you reframe these hurdles as opportunities to shift from a practitioner mindset to a strategic thinker mindset. Let's tackle these hurdles one by one, with practical tools and stories to show you that you *are* proof of what's possible.

HURDLE #1: FORMAL MANAGEMENT TRAINING NOT INCLUDED

There is a false belief that having no formal management training means you are not cut out for leadership. It's true that most physicians do not receive any formal business or leadership training during medical school. Believing that formal management training is required can trigger imposter syndrome. In reality, the very process of becoming a physician—or any other clinician—develops core leadership characteristics. It requires drive, stamina, communication skills, and leadership. We are already practicing critical thinking, making decisions under pressure, and working in teams. Inherently, as a physician, people around you already see you as a leader and authority figure. There will just be a few more skills you will need to acquire to successfully transition from being a patient care leader to a healthcare organizational leader. I have conquered the leadership landscape without the MBA, and I can help you accelerate your leadership journey as well.

The **Dr. Maia Leadership Framework** allows you to reframe that mindset. It will help you reflect on the areas in your personal and professional life where you have been in that leadership role, and you will build on that experience. You will discover that you have what it takes to be successful with the formal training already attained.

Organizational leadership skills can be developed through coaching and practice. There are three key areas that are critical for success that my methodology will ensure you develop: leading dynamic teams, solving problems head-on, and leveraging your emotional intelligence. Just like medicine, learning is lifelong and continuous. It's not about perfection but rather growth.

SELF-ASSESSMENT: READINESS FOR LEADERSHIP

For each question, rate yourself from 1 to 5:

1 = Strongly Disagree | 5 = Strongly Agree

- I make critical decisions under pressure on a regular basis.
- I regularly lead or coordinate care among a team of professionals.
- Colleagues come to me for guidance, mentorship, or second opinions.
- I can clearly and effectively communicate complex information to different audiences (e.g., patients, families, other healthcare providers).
- I take initiative to solve problems or improve processes in my clinical environment.

SCORING

- **5–10: Time to Shift Your Lens**: You may be underestimating your leadership experience. Reflect on the roles you already play—you likely lead more than you realize.
- **11–15: Solid Foundation, Room to Grow**: You show potential and may benefit from guided coaching or strategic exposure to leadership tools.
- **16–20: Leadership-Ready With Momentum**: You have strong leadership instincts. A few targeted skills or frameworks will take you to the next level.
- **21–25: Natural Leader in the Making**: You already exhibit key leadership qualities. You don't need a formal degree—you need refinement, mentorship, and opportunity.

Are You Ready to Counter Your Belief That You Must Have Formal Management Training to Be a Successful Organizational Leader? Make a list of your characteristics and skills that you already have cultivated as a clinician.

MY STORY: FROM IMPOSTER TO INFLUENCER

When I first stepped into leadership, I was terrified I'd be exposed as someone who just simply wasn't ready. I didn't have an MBA, and the boardroom felt like a foreign country where I didn't speak the language. I remember sitting in a meeting, hearing terms like strategic alignment and resource allocation and feeling like I was drowning. But then I realized something: Every time I led a code blue or coordinated a patient's care plan,

I was already making high-stakes decisions and leading teams. I just needed to translate those skills to the organizational level. With the help of a mentor who saw my potential, I started reading leadership books, attending webinars, and practicing new skills like facilitating meetings. Within months, I was leading discussions with confidence, proving that you don't need a business degree. You need determination.

Actionable Takeaway for You: Write down three leadership skills you already use in your clinical work (e.g., decision-making, team coordination, communication). Then, identify one resource—like a book, podcast, or professional organization—that can help you refine one of those skills for organizational leadership. Commit to engaging with that resource this week.

HURDLE #2: WHO HAS TIME TO LEAD?

You think you don't have time for leadership responsibilities. Sometimes when we look at the leaders around us, it appears like endless paperwork, meetings, slow negotiations, and long days and evenings that seem to have little or no impact. We as clinicians already have demanding schedules and really don't need the burden of taking on anything else. Currently, some of us barely have time for our families and personal lives.

My trailblazing insight will help you learn how to prioritize the organizational work and delegate appropriately. Which tasks are absolutely necessary for you, and which tasks can other team members do that will help them grow? Leading effective teams with clear accountability, roles, and responsibilities can go a long way. Ensuring the right balance of clinical and administrative time is critical. This may need to be adjusted over time. My coaching will ensure that you find a leadership role that honors your personal time. A job that requires an hour commute in traffic to and from work may not be suitable for someone who has to pick up their children at a particular time after work.

SELF-ASSESSMENT: LEADERSHIP ALIGNMENT

Rate each statement from 1 to 5:

1 = Strongly Disagree | 5 = Strongly Agree

- I feel like there's room in my schedule for things beyond clinical care.
- I believe that leadership roles do not mean mandatory sacrificing of personal time or family responsibilities.
- I find ease in delegating tasks to others when they are capable.
- I see leadership as less about meetings and bureaucracy and more about impact.
- I intentionally build in time to mentor or empower others on my team.
- I know what tasks only I can do—and which ones I could delegate.
- I have clarity around what type of leadership role would align with my life outside of medicine.

SCORING

- **7–14: Time-Pressed Skeptic**: You may be feeling maxed out or unclear about what leadership really looks like.

With some mindset shifts and structural strategies, leadership can be realistic—and even energizing.

- **15–24: Balancing Act in Progress**: You're juggling a lot, but you're starting to see where leadership might fit. With intentional support and boundaries, you can grow without burnout.
- **25–35: Strategic Time Steward**: You have the mindset and self-awareness to lead effectively. You understand the value of delegation, prioritization, and choosing roles that align with your values.

Think about your mornings, afternoons, evenings, nights, and weekends. Which days and times are you willing to work, and when do you need to ensure your time is spent attending to your personal priorities? In your current workplace, can you see opportunities for more delegation and division of tasks? In which areas can the work become more efficient?

MY STORY: FINDING TIME TO LEAD

I used to think leadership would mean giving up what little personal time I had left. As a mom, my evenings were sacred—dinner with my kids, bedtime stories, the chaos of family life. But when I took on my first leadership role, I was determined to make it work. I started by auditing my day. I realized I was spending hours on tasks that others could handle, like routine scheduling or data entry. I began delegating those tasks to my team, which not only freed up my time but also empowered them to grow. I also negotiated a schedule that allowed me to leave in time to pick up my children from school. Leadership didn't take time away—it gave me control over my time.

Actionable Takeaway for You: This week, identify one task you're doing that someone else on your team could handle. Delegate it, and use the time you save to focus on a strategic goal—like preparing for a leadership discussion or researching a role that excites you. Delegation is your key to making time for leadership.

HURDLE #3: RED TAPE OVERLOAD

Leadership is too much bureaucracy and red tape. Nothing gets done. I get it, observing a lot of bureaucracy and red tape may deter you from moving into leadership, but it doesn't have to. These challenges are indeed real but do not have to consume your leadership experience. Even as you are just getting started and rounding out your leadership skills, you have to understand your distinct position of influence: your unique duality. You are a well-respected clinician and you are also a leader who is growing into a well-rounded administrator. You will begin to realize that your biggest superpower as an administrator is that you are a clinician first. This duality allows us to have a special influence on the people we are leading in the organization.

As your coach, I will help you tap into this superpower and leverage your unique skills of moving other clinicians through change. Remember, you may likely be one of the few clinicians in the boardroom, and your unique insights and perspectives matter. There will be no one who can influence another clinician as much as a fellow clinician with shared experience.

We will discuss common frustrations and find ways for you to help fix problems. Working together, we will find opportunities for you to leverage your voice and have impact on things like workflows and policies that make sense.

SELF-ASSESSMENT: LEADING BEYOND RED TAPE

Rate each statement from 1 to 5:

1 = Strongly Disagree | 5 = Strongly Agree

- I believe that healthcare leadership red tape does not have to slow down progress.
- Leaders rarely struggle to implement change due to administrative hurdles.
- I feel like my ideas for improvement rarely get lost in the system.
- Being a clinician gives me insight that many administrators do not have.
- I've used my clinical experience to influence decisions beyond direct patient care.
- I can see how clinician-leaders are uniquely positioned to bridge the gap between the bedside and the boardroom.

SCORING

- **6–12: Red Tape Resister**: You may be feeling stuck before you've even started. You're likely focusing on what doesn't work in leadership—without seeing how your clinician voice can cut through the noise.

- **13–21: Emerging Bridge Builder**: You understand the tension between clinical work and bureaucracy, and you're starting to see how your perspective can create change. With targeted coaching, this duality becomes a major asset.
- **22–30: Clinician Change Agent**: You already recognize your unique power as a clinician-leader. You're well-positioned to navigate bureaucracy strategically and lead with both credibility and clarity.

Do You Want to Stay in the Current Broken System and Suffer or Have a Role in Fixing the System? Why? Are You Letting Bureaucracy Block Your Leadership Potential?

MY STORY: CUTTING THROUGH THE RED TAPE

Early in my leadership journey, I was frustrated by a policy that required clinicians to complete redundant forms, slowing down patient care. I could have stayed silent, assuming the bureaucracy was too big to tackle. Instead, I used my clinician's perspective to propose a streamlined workflow at a leadership meeting. I was nervous, but I framed it as a patient-centered solution, and to my surprise, the room listened. That small win showed me that my voice as a clinician could cut through the red tape. Over time, I learned to navigate bureaucracy by building alliances with key stakeholders and focusing on solutions that aligned with organizational goals.

Actionable Takeaway for You: Identify one bureaucratic frustration in your workplace (e.g., a clunky process or policy). Write down one idea to improve it, and share it with a trusted colleague or supervisor this week. Your clinician perspective is your superpower—use it to start small changes.

HURDLE #4: TRADING IN MY STETHOSCOPE?

You have spent so many years refining your patient care skills, and the thought of losing that can be devastating. There is a real fear of being disconnected with patient care and medicine. After years of refining skills, you don't want them to get rusty.

My methodology will help you understand that you will continue to have significant clinical impact, even as a formal leader. Your clinical knowledge will have a domino effect on a larger scale. I will help you shift your mindset around impact: As a practitioner, influence over one patient at a time and now as a leader influence over a multitude of patients. When we uncover your priorities, we will determine if continuing to see patients is truly a priority for you and, if so, what will the division between clinical and administrative work look like. In addition, my approach will direct you to a leadership role that helps you stay connected to the frontline if that is what you desire.

SELF-ASSESSMENT: CLINICIAN AND LEADER IDENTITY

Rate each statement from 1 to 5:

1 = Strongly Disagree | 5 = Strongly Agree

- Stepping into leadership does not mean giving up the clinical skills I've worked hard to master.

- I can find fulfillment and identity in direct patient care and leadership.
- I do not fear feeling disconnected from the front lines of medicine.
- I've seen clinician-leaders stay clinically active while also influencing organizational decisions.
- I believe that improving systems and teams can impact more patients than I can see individually.
- I can feel confident about leadership while maintaining some clinical responsibilities.
- I see leadership as an extension—not a replacement—of my medical purpose.

SCORING

- **7–14: Clinician at a Crossroads**: You may be feeling conflicted about letting go of direct patient care. It's important to remember leadership can be added to your identity, not traded for it.
- **15–24: Blending Both Worlds**: You're aware of the tension between clinical work and leadership, but you're open to finding a blend that fits. You're on your way to redefining your role with intention.
- **25–35: Purpose-Driven Leader**: You've reframed leadership as a broader form of healing. You recognize that influence isn't limited to exam rooms—and your impact can scale through smart leadership.

How Important Is Having Patient Care Time in Your New Role? What Ways Do You Want to Stay Connected to Medicine? Can You Lead Without Losing Your Clinical Identity?

MY STORY: KEEPING MY STETHOSCOPE CLOSE

I'll never forget the day I realized I could be a leader *and* stay connected to patients. Early in my leadership role, I worried I'd lose the part of me that loved bedside care. So, I negotiated to keep one day a week in the clinic. That time with patients recharged me and informed my leadership decisions. When I proposed a new triage system, it came from my direct experience seeing how delays affected patients. My clinical work didn't just keep my skills sharp—it made me a better leader.

Actionable Takeaway for You: Reflect on how much clinical time you want in your ideal leadership role. Write down one way you could stay connected to patient care (e.g., a weekly clinic day, mentoring residents). Then, research one leadership role that allows for clinical involvement to see what's possible.

HURDLE #5: MANAGING THE MASTERS OF THE CRAFT

Going from being a peer to managing your peers is very awkward. It can be hard to digest the reality of shifting power dynamics. Leadership requires decisions that may impact colleagues' work. As the relationship changes, real concerns about isolation and going without camaraderie can emerge.

My coaching techniques will help you uncover ways to cultivate an even stronger camaraderie by being an advocate. They will count on you to be the voice in the room that understands their concerns. You will be in a position to have influence over what work looks like for your fellow clinicians. My insight will allow you to solve problems and manage conflict.

SELF-ASSESSMENT: LEADING CLINICIAN PEERS

Rate each statement from 1 to 5:

1 = Strongly Disagree | 5 = Strongly Agree

- The idea of leading my current peers does not feel uncomfortable or awkward.
- I rarely worry that stepping into leadership will change how colleagues relate to me.
- I find ease in giving feedback or holding peers accountable without damaging relationships.
- I value professional camaraderie and do not fear losing it if I'm seen as "management."
- I believe it's possible to lead with both authority and humility.
- I'm learning how to separate personal relationships from professional responsibilities when necessary.

SCORING

- **6–12: Reluctant Riser**: You're likely feeling hesitant about managing peers—concerned about losing connection or facing resistance. With guidance, you can grow into a respected and relational leader.

- **13–21: Evolving Leader**: You're aware of the emotional complexities but willing to navigate them. You're building emotional intelligence, trust, and the skills to lead with empathy and clarity.
- **22–30: Grounded Authority**: You've started embracing the shift from peer to leader. You're ready to lead respectfully, hold boundaries, and still foster connection.

Are You Ready to Lead Your Peers With Confidence? What Would It Be Like for You to Finally Advocate and Come Up With Solutions That Not Only Benefit the Organization but Also Clinicians, Thus Gaining You Even More Respect as Not Only a Great Clinician but Also a Great Organizational Leader?

MY STORY: FROM PEER TO PARTNER

Managing my peers was one of my biggest fears. I remember the first time I had to give feedback to a colleague I'd worked with for years. My palms were sweaty, and I worried she'd see me as "the boss" instead of a friend. But I approached it with empathy, framing the feedback as a way to support her growth and improve patient care. To my surprise, she thanked me. That moment taught me that leading peers isn't about power—it's about partnership. By advocating for their needs in leadership meetings, I built stronger bonds than ever.

Actionable Takeaway for You: Practice giving constructive feedback to a colleague this week. Frame it as a collaborative conversation, focusing on a shared goal (e.g., improving patient outcomes). This will build your confidence in leading peers with empathy and authority.

YOUR PATH FORWARD: LEAP OVER THE HURDLES

If you're feeling stuck behind these hurdles, let me remind you: *You are proof.* You're proof that the skills you've honed as a clinician—problem-solving, empathy, resilience—can carry you over these obstacles. The mindset shift from practitioner to strategic thinker is about seeing challenges as opportunities to grow, not barriers to success. My **Dr. Maia Leadership Framework** will guide you through each hurdle, showing you how to leverage your unique strengths as a clinician to become a transformative leader.

Your First Step: Pick one hurdle from this chapter that resonates most with you. Write down one small action you can take this week to address it. Maybe it's listing your leadership skills, delegating a task, proposing a small change to a process, defining your clinical priorities, or practicing feedback with a peer. Whatever it is, take that step. It's the first leap toward your leadership journey.

In the chapters ahead, we'll dive deeper into the **Dr. Maia Leadership Framework**, exploring how to build your **Leadership Arsenal**, how to cultivate strategic relationships, and how to lead with confidence. You'll hear more stories of clinicians who've overcome these hurdles to create meaningful change. Most importantly, you'll discover that leadership isn't about being fearless—it's about being bold enough to try.

CHAPTER 4

The Mindset Shift From Practitioner to Strategic Leader

The secret to becoming a powerful clinician-leader is not found in a new degree or a corner office—it begins with a shift in mindset. To lead effectively, you must transition from identifying solely as a practitioner to embodying the identity of a strategic organizational leader. This transformation is your key to lasting influence. Most clinicians are trained to *do*. We fix, we treat, we manage the immediate. But leadership demands something radically different. It requires you to step out of the weeds and into the role of a visionary. You cannot lead while drowning in tasks. You must delegate to elevate.

This mindset shift is not just a subtle tweak in perspective—it's a seismic reorientation of how you see yourself and your role in the world of healthcare. As a clinician, you've spent years honing your ability to diagnose, treat, and care for patients with precision and compassion. That's your foundation, and it's rock-solid. But to become a leader who shapes systems, influences policy, and drives organizational change, you must build on that foundation with a new identity: one that sees the big picture, anticipates challenges, and inspires others to act. This is where your journey to strategic excellence begins.

Let me share a story to illustrate this shift. Dr. Jordan, a seasoned physician, was known for her meticulous care and ability to connect with patients. She thrived in the exam room, solving problems one at a time. But when she was promoted to lead the clinic, she found herself overwhelmed. She was still trying to manage every patient case herself, review every chart, be the gap provider when other doctors would call in sick, and even handle scheduling conflicts. She was drowning in the weeds, and her team was disengaged because she didn't trust them to take ownership.

One day, a mentor pulled her aside and said, "Dr. Jordan, you're not the doctor in the room anymore. You're the doctor who builds the system so every room runs better." That was her wake-up call. She became more intentional about delegating, empowering her team, and focusing on strategic priorities like improving patient flow and staff training. Within a year, her department's outcomes improved, and she was invited to the executive table to share her insights. Dr. Jordan's transformation wasn't about earning an MBA—it was about embracing her role as a strategic leader.

You will need to move away from being the one doing all of the tasks. If you do not delegate, your leadership journey will fail, because you will get caught up in the weeds and lose vision of where you are going. You will need to learn how to empower those who work for you and trust them to do their job. In doing so, you carve out the mental and emotional space needed to own your role as a leader and drive your organization forward.

Delegation, a key skill in the **Leadership Arsenal**, is not about abandoning your clinical instincts or relinquishing control—it's about amplifying your impact. Imagine trying to perform every role in a hospital: the surgeon, the nurse, the administrator, the janitor. It's impossible, and it's not your job. Your job as a clinician-leader is to create systems where everyone thrives. This means trusting your team to execute while you focus on the bigger picture—whether that's improving patient outcomes, streamlining operations, or advocating for policy changes. To do this, you must release the need to control every detail and embrace the power of collaboration.

Let's break this down into a practical tool you can use today: **The Delegation Blueprint**. Start by identifying tasks that don't require your unique expertise. Ask yourself: "Is this something only I can do, or can someone else handle it with the right guidance?" Create a list of tasks you can delegate—scheduling, routine follow-ups, or data entry, for example. Next, identify the right person for each task based on their strengths. Provide clear instructions, set expectations, and give them the autonomy to execute. Check in periodically, but don't micromanage. Finally, reflect on the time you've freed up and redirect it toward strategic priorities—perhaps analyzing patient data trends or preparing for a leadership meeting. This blueprint doesn't just lighten your load; it builds a culture of trust and empowerment that elevates your entire team.

You must believe in yourself as a **change agent**, a clinician that comes with valuable leadership tools without a formal business education. You have acquired and refined experience, character traits, and critical thinking that enable you to take up space and rise. You have to know that as a clinician leader, you have a superpower of understanding firsthand what quality care looks like and how it is operationalized. Many of your colleagues at the leadership table will not be clinicians and will never understand the role to the extent that you do.

Here's the truth no one told you in med school: You are already a change agent. You don't need an MBA to lead. You've already developed the discipline, resilience, emotional intelligence, and critical thinking required for executive impact—qualities forged in the crucible of clinical care. What you may lack in formal business training can be bridged with the right tools, resources, and strategic relationships.

Think about the skills you've already mastered. As a clinician, you've navigated high-stakes decisions under pressure, communicated with empathy to distressed patients, and solved complex problems with limited information. These are the same skills that make exceptional leaders. The difference lies in how you apply them.

Instead of solving one patient's problem, you're now solving systemic problems. Instead of comforting one family, you're inspiring an entire organization. Your clinical experience is your competitive edge—it's the lens through which you see what others in the boardroom cannot.

To make this mindset shift tangible, try this exercise: **The Leadership Identity Journal**. For the next seven days, write down one moment each day where you acted as a leader, not just a practitioner. Maybe you advocated for a process change, mentored a colleague, or proposed a solution to a systemic issue. Reflect on how it felt to step into that role. What fears did you overcome? What impact did you make? This exercise rewires your brain to see yourself as a leader and not just a clinician. It's a small step with profound results.

As a clinician, you possess a superpower most boardroom peers do not—you understand, intuitively and experientially, what high-quality care looks like and how it's delivered at the ground level. You know what happens when systems fail patients. That insight alone makes you indispensable at the leadership table. Yes, there are gaps—but they are smaller than you think. And with the right coaching, a strong network, and a commitment to growth, those gaps disappear quickly. You are not a "future leader"—you are a leader now. The moment you embrace this mindset shift is the moment you stop waiting for permission and start transforming the systems that need your voice the most.

Consider Dr. James, a clinical outpatient medicine leader. Initially, he felt out of place among the administrators. But during a discussion about improving processes in access to specialty care, he shared a vivid example of how a poorly designed process led to a patient's delay in care. His story grounded the conversation in reality, shifting the focus from abstract metrics to patient impact. The room listened. His perspective didn't just influence the decision—it reshaped the hospital's entire approach to triage. Dr. James didn't need a business degree to make that impact; he needed the confidence to own his unique value.

To bridge any gaps in your leadership toolkit, seek out three key resources: **coaching**, **networks**, and **continuous learning**. A coach can help you refine your strategic thinking and navigate organizational dynamics. A network of fellow clinician-leaders provides support, ideas, and opportunities to collaborate. And continuous learning—through books, webinars, or even online courses—equips you with the business acumen to complement your clinical expertise.

Start small: Join a professional organization like the American College of Healthcare Executives, attend a leadership workshop, or find a mentor who's walked this path. These steps don't require a degree, but they do require commitment.

You will know the shift has occurred when you voice your unique perspective at the decision table and realize your perspective elevates the conversation to an entirely new level. Your mindset shift will show up in your confident tone, demeanor, and walk. It's important to not be overconfident or overly assertive at the decision-making table. You will need to be recognized as a leader who listens, collaborates, and empowers others. You walk in humility and with the willingness to learn and grow. If you find yourself walking away from the table without a clear understanding of how your message has resonated with others, or if you find you are unclear about the perspectives of others in the room, this may be a clue that you have not yet found the balance between your confident voice and being overconfident.

This balance is critical. Confidence without humility can alienate colleagues and stifle collaboration. Humility without confidence can make you invisible at the table. To find this balance, practice **active listening** and **reflective questioning**. When you're at the decision table, listen intently to others' perspectives before sharing your own. Ask questions like: "Can you clarify how this impacts patient care?" or "What challenges do you foresee in implementing this?" These questions show you value others' input while positioning you to share your insights thoughtfully. After the meeting, reflect: Did you contribute meaningfully? Did you understand the room's dynamics? This practice sharpens your ability to lead with both authority and empathy.

Active listening and reflective questioning are powerful tools for cultivating the balance of confidence and humility in professional settings. Active listening involves fully engaging with the speaker, maintaining eye contact, nodding to acknowledge understanding, and avoiding interruptions or distractions. It means absorbing not just the words but the intent and emotions behind them, which builds trust and demonstrates respect for colleagues' perspectives. Reflective questioning complements this by prompting deeper exploration of ideas without asserting dominance.

For example, asking "Can you elaborate on how this approach aligns with our long-term goals?" or "What assumptions are we making here?" invites clarification and encourages collaborative problem-solving. These techniques ensure you're not just heard but also valued as a thoughtful contributor who elevates the conversation while fostering inclusivity.

Let's wrap this up with a challenge: **The 30-Day Leadership Shift Challenge**. For the next 30 days, commit to one daily action that reinforces your identity as a strategic leader. It could be delegating a task, sharing an idea in a meeting, or reaching out to a mentor. Track your progress in a journal, noting how each action makes you feel and the impact it has. By the end of the challenge, you'll not only feel like a leader—you'll be leading. Your team will notice, your organization will benefit, and you'll prove to yourself that you are, indeed, proof of what's possible.

This mindset shift is your gateway to strategic excellence. It's not about abandoning your clinical roots; it's about leveraging them to create systemic change. You are not just a clinician. You are a visionary, a change agent, and a leader. Own it. The systems you serve and the patients who depend on them are waiting for your voice.

CHAPTER 5

Embracing Leadership—Overcoming Isolation and Self-Doubt

You could be thinking to yourself that you are somehow different. You could be thinking that you are in a special circumstance and that leadership just cannot work for you. You might even be feeling isolated and alone. There are several common scenarios that may fit your circumstance. You may have applied for leadership roles in the past and you didn't get the jobs. Or perhaps you are a seasoned clinician, and you were asked to fill a leadership vacancy. In this instance, you may have been thrust in with no orientation. You were just left alone and expected to pick up where the last person left off.

Whatever your reason, you have not been successful, and it has not worked out. Perhaps you feel disconnected and lonely or that there is something others have that you don't. You may have even had coaching that focused on the fundamental business acumen of management and leadership, likely sitting alongside your clinician peers. And yet all of that leadership preparation is not kicking in. You still feel like an outsider, scared to make a mistake, and all alone. There could be a lot of shame or self-doubt.

If this sounds like you, then you are in good company. All of these feelings are very common, and I personally know what it means to flounder publicly and want to literally run away and hide or secretly find a reason to return to full-time patient care, because that was a cakewalk compared to the new and different leadership terrain. However, it's so worth it. You must persevere and remember the impact you can make with both patients and staff, streamlining operations, and your voice in affecting healthcare policy.

Let's pause and acknowledge the weight of those feelings. Isolation and self-doubt are not signs of failure—they're part of the human experience, especially when stepping into the uncharted territory of leadership. As clinicians, we're trained to project confidence and competence, but leadership exposes vulnerabilities we may not have faced in the exam room. The good news? These feelings are not roadblocks; they're signposts pointing you toward growth. The moment you recognize and confront them is the moment you begin to transform.

Consider this: every clinician-leader who's made an impact has faced these same doubts. I've been there myself and so have countless others. Let me share a story to bring this home. Maria, a brilliant Nurse Leader, was tapped to lead her hospital's quality improvement initiative. She was thrilled at the opportunity but soon felt out of her depth. Meetings with executives left her second-guessing her contributions, and she felt like an imposter among seasoned administrators. She confided in me, "I'm used to saving lives, not leading meetings. I feel like I'm failing at this."

Through coaching, Maria learned to reframe her self-doubt as a signal to seek support and build relationships. She started connecting with colleagues, asking questions, and sharing her clinical insights in a way that bridged the gap between patient care and strategy. Within months, she was leading with confidence, and her initiative reduced readmission rates significantly. Maria's breakthrough wasn't about erasing doubt—it was about using it as fuel to grow.

My **Dr. Maia Leadership Framework** will walk you through this process at your own pace and is customized just for you. You will address the internal work to help you believe in yourself, get clear on your personal priorities, and walk boldly along a career trajectory that is best suited for you. We take our time to understand what a meaningful, fulfilling life looks like to you. Then, we craft a customized plan for you to accomplish your goals quickly. We will go into more detail on this road map in chapter 7.

This program is designed to meet you where you are. It's not a one-size-fits-all approach—it's a personalized journey that acknowledges your unique challenges and strengths. Whether you're grappling with rejection from past leadership applications or feeling abandoned in a new role, my **Dr. Maia Leadership Framework** helps you break through the isolation and build a foundation for success. It's about more than skills; it's about rediscovering your purpose and aligning it with your leadership path.

Let's talk about a practical tool to combat isolation and self-doubt: **The Connection Compass.** This exercise helps you map out your support network and leverage it to thrive as a leader. Step one: List five people in your professional or personal life who can support your leadership journey—a mentor, a peer, a coach, a friend, or even a family member. Step two: Reach out to one of them each week for a meaningful conversation. Ask for advice, share a challenge, or simply listen to their perspective. Step three: Reflect on how these connections make you feel less alone and more empowered. This compass doesn't just build relationships—it builds your confidence to show up authentically at the leadership table.

I can think of a leader who gladly stepped up to fulfill a high turnover role but was soon challenged with competing personal priorities. Dr. Lisa was honored to take on a supervisory role, and she prided herself on her love for finding solutions for better patient flow. She was a team player and wanted to support her executive leadership by filling a gap in their fleet of supervisors. She had a great reputation as a clinician and could be counted on to take care of patients extremely well, earning amazing patient satisfaction scores.

It wasn't long before her gusto for having an impact waned due to too much time away from home. Her spouse often complained about not having enough quality time at home as she was spending late hours in her office. Disappointment emerged after being let down time and time again with her ideas being not accepted. She had not tapped into the fact that she worked in an ecosystem and not in isolation. She failed to build relationships, and her communication approach was not good. She had the title but was left feeling miserable daily.

Dr. Lisa's story is a powerful reminder that leadership isn't just about stepping up—it's about staying connected. Her isolation stemmed from a lack of relationships within her organization and a failure to align her role with her personal priorities. She was trying to do it all alone, and that's a recipe for burnout. The turning point came when she joined a peer mentoring group for clinician-leaders. Through candid discussions, she realized her communication style—direct and clinical—wasn't resonating with her administrative colleagues.

She learned to frame her ideas in terms of organizational goals, build alliances with key stakeholders, and set boundaries to protect her family time. Within six months, her ideas were gaining traction, and she felt reinvigorated. Dr. Lisa didn't need to change who she was—she needed to connect and communicate strategically.

To avoid Dr. Lisa's early struggles, embrace this principle: **Leadership is a team sport**. You don't succeed by going it alone. You succeed by building a network of allies who amplify your voice and share your vision. Start by identifying one person in your organization whose perspective you respect. Invite them for coffee or a virtual chat. Ask about their challenges and share one of yours. This small act of connection can open doors to collaboration and support, making you feel less like an outsider and more like a vital part of the ecosystem.

The first few weeks in my first leadership job, I felt isolated, overwhelmed, and scared. What was missing was a coach who was by my side, helping me create a customized road map and providing consistent support and coaching through my early challenges for timely navigation of this new leadership territory.

That's one of the many reasons I've created this program for you—I know what I needed way back then, and I'm offering it to you now.

That personal experience shaped my mission to ensure no clinician-leader feels alone. I remember sitting in my office, staring at a stack of reports, wondering if I'd made a mistake leaving full-time patient care. The turning point came when I found a mentor who saw my potential and helped me see it too. She didn't just teach me skills—she helped me reframe my fears as opportunities. That's what the **Dr. Maia Leadership Framework** does for you. It's the coach I wish I'd had, offering you a safe space to process doubts, clarify your goals, and build a road map that's as unique as you are.

Here's another tool to overcome self-doubt: **The Confidence Anchor Exercise**. Identify a moment in your clinical career when you felt unstoppable—maybe a time you saved a patient's life or solved a complex case. Write down every detail: how it felt, what you did, and why it mattered. This is your anchor. When self-doubt creeps in, revisit this moment to remind yourself of your resilience and capability. Then, ask yourself, "If I could do that, what's stopping me from leading with the same strength?" This exercise grounds you in your proven ability to overcome challenges, shifting your mindset from fear to empowerment.

Let's end with another challenge to put this into action that complements the **30-Day Leadership Shift Challenge**: **The 30-Day Connection Challenge**. For the next 30 days, commit to one small act of connection each day. It could be sending a thank-you email to a colleague, asking a question in a meeting, or scheduling a check-in with a mentor. Track these actions in a journal, noting how they make you feel and how others respond. By the end of the challenge, you'll have built a web of relationships that makes isolation a thing of the past. You'll also notice your self-doubt fading as you see the impact of your voice.

You are not alone, and you are not inadequate. The feelings of isolation and self-doubt are part of the journey, but they don't define it. You have the power to rise above them by connecting with others, leaning on support, and anchoring yourself in your strengths. Leadership isn't about being fearless—it's about moving forward despite fear. With the right tools, community, and mindset, you'll not only survive this new terrain—you'll thrive in it, proving to yourself and others that you are ready to lead now.

CHAPTER 6

Embracing Your Leadership Potential

The main focus of this **Dr. Maia Leadership Framework** is to ensure that your personal vision remains at the forefront of your actions. No one is going to believe in you or follow you as a leader if you don't believe in yourself first. Dress like a leader, speak like a leader, move like a leader. Go to events and meet other leaders; join organizations where you are amongst other leaders. Decide that the time is now to make a move to accomplish your goal. Now is the time to step into your true gifts and talents unapologetically. You will need to reframe your mindset around not seeing a full load of patients like you have done for years. The shift will move from measuring success by individualized clinical excellence to measuring success by your ability to improve delivery of care, team performance, and finding solutions to impact organizational goals. Your performance will be indicated by patient outcomes, patient satisfaction surveys, productivity, and strategic initiatives.

This shift begins with the foundation by creating a clear career vision, exploring your skills, and identifying your personal priorities. Your career vision is the North Star guiding your leadership journey—perhaps you see yourself as a medical director streamlining care delivery or a policy influencer shaping equitable healthcare systems. You explored your skills, recognizing strengths like critical thinking and empathy, while identifying gaps, such as data analysis or team management, that you're ready to bridge. Most importantly, you clarified your personal priorities—time with family, personal wellness, or professional growth—that ensure your leadership aligns with your life's non-negotiables. This foundation is the bedrock of your transformation, grounding every step you take in this chapter as you embrace your leadership potential.

This shift in mindset is both liberating and challenging. As a clinician, you've spent years defining your value through direct patient care—every diagnosis, every treatment plan, and every life touched. That's your comfort zone, and it's where you've thrived. But leadership asks you to redefine success, to measure your impact not by the patients you see in a day but by the systems you improve, the teams you inspire, and the policies you shape. This doesn't mean abandoning your clinical roots; it means leveraging them to create exponential impact. You're no longer just healing individuals—you're healing healthcare itself.

Let's bring this to life with a story. Dr. Logan, an internist with a stellar reputation, was hesitant to step into a leadership role. He loved his patient interactions and feared losing that connection. But when his hospital needed a director for its primary care network, he felt a pull to contribute on a larger scale. Initially, he struggled to let go of his clinical identity. He kept jumping into patient care tasks, leaving little time for strategic planning. Through mentorship, he learned to delegate clinical duties and focus on initiatives like reducing wait times and improving care coordination. Within a year, his network's patient satisfaction scores soared, and he found a new sense of purpose. Dr. Logan's transformation wasn't about leaving patient care behind—it was about embracing a broader vision of impact.

Dr. Logan's journey began with the foundational work. He clarified his career vision: to lead a network that delivered seamless, patient-centered care. He assessed his skills, leaning on his strength in building rapport while committing to learning data-driven decision-making. His personal priorities—maintaining work-life balance and mentoring young clinicians—shaped his leadership approach, ensuring he delegated tasks to protect his time. By grounding his actions in this foundation, Dr. Logan turned his hesitation into impact, proving that a clear vision, skill awareness, and aligned priorities are the springboard to leadership success.

Now is the time to build a community around you, so you can be like a sponge and acquire new skills and knowledge to transition from clinical excellence to organizational excellence. You will get stronger daily as you stop becoming the taskmaster. You will hire, orient, and coach your direct reports on the tasks you want them to do. This is critical. No more in the weeds for you. You are used to being the most educated person in the room. You have to be okay with being in spaces where you have the most to learn in the room.

This community building ties directly emphasis on vision and priorities. Your career vision guides who you connect with—mentors who've achieved what you aspire to, peers who share your goals, and mentees who energize your purpose. Your skills exploration helps you identify gaps to address through these connections, like learning strategic planning from a mentor. Your personal priorities ensure your community respects your boundaries, such as protecting family time while growing professionally. By aligning your community, you create a support system that amplifies your leadership potential.

Building this community is like constructing a bridge to your leadership potential. You can't cross the gap from practitioner to strategic leader alone—you need allies, mentors, and peers who challenge and support you. Think of it as creating your own leadership ecosystem. This community will expose you to new ideas, help you navigate organizational dynamics, and remind you that you're not alone in this journey. It's about surrounding yourself with people who see your potential, even when you doubt it yourself.

Here's a practical tool to get started: **The Leadership Circle Builder**. Identify three types of connections to cultivate: a mentor who's ahead of you in their leadership journey, a peer who's navigating similar challenges, and a mentee you can guide. Reach out to one person in each category within the next week. Schedule a conversation to share your goals and ask for their insights. For example, ask your mentor, "What helped you transition from clinical to strategic leadership?" or ask your peer, "How do you balance clinical and administrative demands?" These connections will not only provide knowledge but also reinforce your commitment to growth.

Revisit your career vision before reaching out. For instance, if your vision is to lead a quality improvement initiative, seek a mentor who's done that. If a priority is work-life balance, ask your peer how they manage it. This alignment ensures your community supports your foundational goals, making your leadership circle a powerful catalyst for transformation.

I joined a national healthcare leadership organization to gain the tools I needed to manage people and understand strategy. I invested in reputable magazines, webinars, and conferences. I felt out of place and often the only doctor in a room full of formally trained administrators, but I worked through those sensations and learned leadership techniques and information I needed in order to swim.

That was a turning point for me. I remember walking into my first conference, feeling like an imposter among suits and MBAs. But I pushed through, asked questions, and absorbed everything I could. One conversation with a seasoned administrator gave me a framework for aligning clinical goals with organizational strategy—a game-changer.

That's the power of stepping into spaces where you're not the expert. It's humbling, but it's also where growth happens. You don't need to know everything—you just need to be willing to learn.

My career vision—to influence healthcare systems—drove me to join that organization. Exploring my skills showed me

I needed to learn strategic communication, which I sought through webinars. My priority of personal growth pushed me to attend conferences despite discomfort. By connecting these actions to my foundation, I turned fear into opportunity. You can do the same by ensuring each step aligns with your vision and priorities.

To make this actionable, try **The Learning Leap Strategy**. Commit to one new learning opportunity each month—a webinar, a leadership book, or a conference session. Before you engage, write down one specific skill or insight you want to gain, like "how to lead effective meetings" or "strategies for team motivation." After the experience, reflect on how you can apply what you learned. This strategy turns passive learning into active growth, helping you build confidence and competence.

Are you ready for your transformation? Despite the doubts and fears, there was no turning back for me. I felt something pulling me toward this new leadership trajectory. I held the vision of myself as a great impactful leader in my head. I wanted to be a great leader with the same fervor I had to be a great clinician.

This pull is your inner compass, guiding you toward a purpose bigger than yourself. It's not about ego—it's about impact. You're not just leading for the title; you're leading to make healthcare better, to empower your team, and to serve patients on a systemic level. That vision is what will carry you through moments of doubt. Hold it close, and let it fuel your determination.

Career vision amplifies this compass. If you envisioned leading a department, let that image drive your actions—join a leadership group or pitch an initiative. If your priority is mentoring others, focus on building relationships that allow you to guide and inspire. You ensure your leadership journey is authentic and sustainable.

Let's pause and do a brief exercise. Ask yourself:

What is your why? What is the reason for continuing the path of clinician leadership?

____

____

What is the risk of not moving forward with your leadership journey?

____

____

If you move forward with your leadership journey, what good may happen?

____

____

Complete this statement:

I am ready for a transformation and want more __________ ______________________________ and the risk is too high to stay in my current role. It's costing me __________________ _______________ and I must move now.

This exercise is a wake-up call. It forces you to confront the cost of staying still—missed opportunities, unfulfilled potential, and a healthcare system that needs your voice. Your *why* is your anchor, and the risks of inaction are your motivation. Revisit these answers whenever you feel stuck. They'll remind you why this journey matters.

Frame your *why* around your career vision. For example, if your vision is to improve patient access, your *why* might be "to ensure every patient receives timely care." If a priority is personal growth, your risk of inaction might be "stagnating in my comfort zone." This alignment makes the exercise more powerful, grounding your motivation in the foundation you've built.

To deepen this reflection, try The Vision Clarity Meditation as you learned in the Introduction of this book. Find a quiet space and spend five minutes visualizing yourself as a confident, impactful leader. Picture yourself leading a meeting, presenting a game-changing idea, or celebrating a team's success. Notice how you feel—confident, energized, purposeful. Write down three words that describe this version of you. Keep them somewhere visible, like your desk or phone, as a daily reminder of who you're becoming.

This meditation builds on career vision.

Use this picture you crafted—perhaps of yourself leading a quality initiative or mentoring a team—as the basis for your visualization. Incorporate your personal priorities, like feeling balanced or fulfilled, to make the image authentic. This practice reinforces your belief in your leadership potential, turning your foundation into a vivid, motivating reality.

I approached the leadership learning curve with the same intensity I put forth in medical school. Back then, I sought resources and subject matter experts to help get me to my goal. Likewise, as my leadership circle of colleagues grew, I began observing their leadership and communication styles. I took the things I liked from them, attributes I saw as missing in my own leadership style. I developed my own approach from what I had learned from watching others. In my **Dr. Maia Leadership Framework**, I will help you reflect on the leaders in your proximity to glean insight as you hone your leadership style. As uncomfortable as it was, I asked for feedback on my presentations and leadership style. I slowly began to create a team of success around me. Each teammate propelled me forward, either professionally, personally, or both.

This process was informed by skill exploration. I identified gaps in my communication style and sought role models to address them. My career vision—to lead with authenticity—guided which traits I adopted, like active listening, while my priority of personal growth pushed me to seek feedback despite discomfort. Let your skill gaps direct you to leaders who excel in those areas, and let your vision shape the style you craft. In my **Dr. Maia Leadership Framework,** I'll guide you through this process, helping you curate a leadership approach that's uniquely yours.

Here's another tool to accelerate this process: **The Feedback Loop Formula**. After every significant interaction—whether it's a presentation, meeting, or one-on-one—ask one trusted colleague for specific feedback. Use this prompt: "What's one thing I did well and one thing I could improve?" Write down their responses and look for patterns over time. This formula turns feedback into a growth engine, helping you refine your style without feeling overwhelmed.

Choose colleagues from your **Leadership Circle Builder** who share your career vision or priorities. For example, if your vision is to improve team performance, ask a mentor who's done that for feedback on your delegation skills. This ensures the feedback supports your foundational goals, accelerating your growth.

Let's wrap up with a challenge to ignite your transformation: **The 30-Day Leadership Presence Challenge**. For the next 30 days, commit to one daily action that reinforces your leadership identity. It could be dressing more confidently, speaking up in a meeting, connecting with a new colleague, or practicing a leadership skill like active listening. Track your actions in a journal, noting how they impact your confidence and how others respond. By the end of the challenge, you'll see tangible evidence of your growth—and you'll feel the shift from clinician to strategic leader.

Ground this challenge by selecting actions that reflect your career vision, skills, and priorities. If your vision is to lead a department, speak up in a strategic meeting. If a priority is wellness, practice a boundary-setting skill. This alignment makes the challenge a powerful extension of your foundation, ensuring your actions are purposeful and impactful.

Embracing your leadership potential is about owning your vision, building your community, and stepping into spaces where you can learn and grow. You're not just a clinician—you're a catalyst for change. The healthcare system needs your voice, your passion, and your unique perspective. Say yes to this journey. The time is now, and you are ready.

Your career, vision, skills, and priorities—is the launchpad for this transformation. It's what makes your leadership authentic and sustainable. Let your vision guide your steps, your skills shape your learning, and your priorities protect your balance. You are proof that clinical excellence can become strategic excellence. Step into it with confidence, and let's make your leadership impact unstoppable. As we get ready for chapter seven, let's learn more about the **Dr. Maia Leadership Framework**.

CHAPTER 7

The Dr. Maia Leadership Framework in Action

STEP 1: TRUST YOUR IDENTITY

You must envision yourself as a leader and see yourself as successful and creating impact. Take time to describe the who, where, and whys of your impact. What area of healthcare are you drawn to? It could be roles like Chief Medical Officer or Chief Innovation Officer. Are you working within a hospital setting or clinic, or are you working remotely? Are you supervising other clinicians or a mix of clinicians and non-clinicians? I love to ask my clients: "In this future you're envisioning, what are you wearing? A business suit or scrubs?" Get excited about this vision of yourself. With your head up and shoulders back, move as though you are already in the position. As you walk into the grocery store, pull up at the gas station, or take your seat at the restaurant, in your mind, you are the organizational leader of your dreams. Folks not only respect you as their leader but also want you as their leader.

This step is about embodying your leadership identity before you even step into the role. Visualization is a powerful tool—athletes use it to win races, and clinicians can use it to win at leadership. Picture yourself leading a boardroom discussion, presenting a transformative idea, or celebrating a team's success. This mental rehearsal rewires your brain to see yourself as a leader, not just a clinician. It's not about pretending—it's about preparing.

Let's bring this to life with a story. Dr. Thomas, a family medicine physician, dreamed of becoming a Chief Medical Officer but felt stuck in his clinical role. He started visualizing himself in that leadership position, imagining himself confidently addressing his team in a suit, not scrubs. He practiced walking with purpose, speaking with authority, and he even attended a leadership networking event to test his new mindset. At first, it felt unnatural, but over time, his confidence grew. When an opportunity arose to lead a quality improvement initiative, he stepped up, leveraging his vision to guide his actions. That role became his stepping stone to a CMO position. Dr. Thomas's transformation began with trusting his identity as a leader before the title was his.

Try this tool to make this step actionable: **The Leadership Vision Board**. Create a physical or digital board with images, words, or quotes that represent your leadership identity. Include symbols of your dream role—perhaps a photo of a hospital boardroom, a leadership quote that inspires you, or even a sketch of yourself in a suit instead of scrubs. Place it somewhere you'll see daily, like on your desk or phone wallpaper. Spend five minutes each morning reflecting on it, asking, "How can I embody this leader today?" This practice keeps your vision front and center, fueling your motivation.

STEP 2: KNOW YOUR STRENGTHS

Take a careful inventory of your strengths. There are several credentialed tools to help you learn more about your strengths and your personality characteristics. Time for another exercise: Think back over the last three months and answer the following questions.

What compliments did you receive?

____

____

Is there a skill or strength that people frequently seem to notice?

____

____

Oftentimes, people have complimented me on my enthusiasm and my ability to give eloquent presentations and find inspiration. These are gifts I project with ease and hardly notice myself. Doing a strength assessment identified my personal strengths of achievement and developing others. Another assessment indicated that those around me view me as nurturing, loyal, and sincere. I have emotional depth, present ideas and concepts with gusto, and quickly build relationships. I share these assessments with my clients. As

I encourage my clients to take these assessments, it's fun to watch their confidence crescendo as these tools uncover talents and uniqueness.

When you are clear on your strengths and natural abilities, you can more clearly align with the leadership role that fits you best and tap into your own unique power to pursue the right opportunities that fit you. You will not fall into positions that, even when you have the technical qualifications, won't enable you to move with ease. You will fully show up powerful and confident. Your colleagues will see how you are uniquely positioned for the job.

Knowing your strengths is like discovering your leadership superpower. As a clinician, you're used to diagnosing patients—now it's time to diagnose yourself. Your strengths are the tools you bring to the leadership table, setting you apart from others. For example, your ability to empathize with patients can translate into inspiring teams. Your knack for problem-solving in the clinic can drive innovative solutions in the boardroom.

To dive deeper, try **The Strength Spotlight Exercise**. Take a strengths assessment like StrengthsFinder or VIA Character Strengths Then, pick one strength and brainstorm three ways to apply it in a leadership context. For instance, if your strength is communication, you might use it to deliver compelling presentations, mediate team conflicts, or advocate for policy changes. Share your findings with a trusted colleague or mentor to gain their perspective. This exercise not only clarifies your strengths but also builds confidence in how they translate to leadership.

Consider Dr. Malik, an anesthesiologist who felt unsure about his leadership potential. A strengths assessment revealed his talents for strategic thinking and building trust. He leaned into these by proposing a new protocol for operating room efficiency, presenting it with data and empathy for his team's workload. His colleagues noticed his unique ability to bridge clinical and strategic goals, earning him a promotion to department chair. Dr. Malik's clarity about his strengths turned uncertainty into impact.

STEP 3: REBOUND FROM SETBACKS

If you are anything like me and many other high-performing clinicians, you do not like to fail; you want everything to be perfect and flawless. The reality is that we are full of imperfections. When I finally learned to embrace my imperfections, life sure got a lot easier, and I could then enjoy the journey. Because the core mechanism for this clinical leadership journey is to believe in yourself, you will need to trust yourself to acquire resources to help you succeed.

With every misstep, you will need to trust that your circle of friends, colleagues, and resources will help you bounce back stronger. It's not easy at all. On those days when I felt like my missteps were winning, I leveraged my tool of exercise to clear my mind and release negativity. I envisioned myself as that strong, impactful leader that I still was, and I decided what adjustments I needed to make.

There was a particular time when a direct report, Charles, gave me feedback on my leadership. I asked him to find out some information. Charles did just that and reported back in an email the same day. I failed to review my email thoroughly, and the next day, I asked for the same information. He expressed how frustrated he was that I failed to check first before asking him again to do the same task. I addressed it with my entire team, apologized, and made a commitment to double-check for a response before re-requesting.

Feeling bad and less than perfect, I took refuge in my circuit training, which is a form of high intensity aerobics, where I could relieve the stress, clear my mind of the self-criticism, and feed myself affirming thoughts like, "You got this, you are growing, you are stronger," "Upward and onward," and "Good job for the transparency you showed your team, and good job for creating a culture where Charles felt comfortable sharing his concerns with you." After an hour of exercise, I found my bounce back, and I went to work the next day with a settled mind.

Setbacks are not failures—they're feedback. As a clinician, you're trained to learn from every patient outcome, adjusting your approach as needed. Leadership is no different. Each misstep is a chance to refine your skills and strengthen your resilience. The key is to reframe setbacks as opportunities to grow, not as evidence of inadequacy.

Here's a tool to help you rebound: **The Setback Recovery Plan**. After a leadership misstep—like a rejected proposal or a team conflict—write down three things: what happened, what you learned, and one action you'll take to move forward. For example, if you receive critical feedback like I did with Charles, your action might be setting a reminder to check emails before assigning tasks. Then, do something to reset your mindset—

exercise, meditate, or talk to a mentor. This plan turns setbacks into stepping stones, keeping you focused on growth.

One of my first major initiatives—a new alternative hours work schedule—failed to gain traction with upper leadership. The executive leadership team resisted, and I felt defeated. Instead of retreating, I sought feedback, learned that my communication lacked clarity, and revised my approach with a focus on buy-in. My second attempt succeeded, and my team praised my adaptability. This rebound wasn't about perfection—it was about persistence and learning.

STEP 4: UNDERSTAND THE ECONOMIC IMPACT

Are you living the life you and your family deserve? Economics impact the life we want to live. Are you making the money and living the life you envisioned upon becoming a clinician? If you are in primary care, my assumption is that your answer might be: "Not exactly." And even if you are a specialist, it's likely that if you have your own practice, the costs associated with that, from the rising costs of insurance to staff and office expenses, mean you are not netting what you envisioned while in medical school.

I've heard from other clinicians that it just took one family diagnosis or a natural disaster to really rock their financial stability. Until I went through a divorce, I didn't anticipate the financial challenges of a divorce or the dynamic costs of raising children for the most part by myself, managing the household, and doing all the day-to-day decision-making without a partner.

I want to create an economic impact for myself, my children, and my community. Economics is a big driving force, and it's important to be clear on how your next chapter will affect your economics. This will impact the life you want to live. We have sacrificed so much, both financially and with time by attaining and maintaining our degrees, medical licenses, and board certifications. The time is now for us to pause and boldly pivot to address our economics.

Leadership roles often come with greater financial rewards and stability, but they also require clarity about your economic goals. Are you seeking a role that maximizes income, provides flexibility, or supports your community? For example, a Chief Medical Officer role might offer a higher salary but demand more hours, while a consulting role could provide flexibility but less predictability. Understanding your economic *why* ensures you pursue opportunities that align with your life vision.

Try this exercise: **The Economic Vision Map**. Write down your ideal financial and lifestyle outcomes five years from now. Include specifics: income, work hours, family time, and community impact. Then, list three leadership roles that could get you there, such as medical director or policy advisor. For each, note one step you can take now—like researching job descriptions or networking with someone in that role. This map keeps your economic goals in focus, guiding your leadership journey.

STEP 5: VALUE YOUR SUCCESS CIRCLE

Creating a close circle of key affirmers, such as mentors, leaders, and friends, is essential for ensuring a focused mindset and achieving sustained success in landing your desired leadership position. This supportive network provides invaluable feedback, encouragement, and insights that help you navigate the complexities of leadership roles.

Imagine having a group of trusted individuals who believe in your potential and are committed to your growth. These key affirmers can offer diverse perspectives, helping you see opportunities and challenges from different angles. Mentors, for instance, can share their experiences and guide you through the intricacies of leadership, while friends and peers can provide emotional support and motivation.

By surrounding yourself with affirmers, you create an environment that fosters resilience and growth. They can help you identify your strengths and areas for improvement, ensuring you are well-prepared for leadership challenges. This network also holds you accountable, pushing you to stay focused on your goals and maintain a positive mindset.

To build this circle, use **The Success Circle Blueprint**. Identify one mentor, one peer, and one friend to include. Schedule a monthly check-in with each, asking for specific feedback or advice on your leadership goals. For example, ask your mentor, "What's one skill I should prioritize to prepare for a CMO role?" or ask your peer, "How do you handle boardroom dynamics?" These connections create a safety net for growth and accountability.

Dr. Nguyen, a surgeon, built a success circle that transformed his career. He connected with a mentor who guided him through hospital politics, a peer who shared strategies for balancing clinical and leadership duties, and a friend who reminded him to celebrate small wins. This circle helped him secure a well-respected leadership role in academic medicine in his healthcare organization. Your success circle is your lifeline—build it intentionally.

STEP 6: EMPOWER YOURSELF WITH RESOURCES

Be clear about where you are on the knowledge barometer. As stated earlier, you have knowledge gaps. When things are new and different, these gaps are big—sometimes big enough to get discouraged very easily. Just like the saying, you can look at the glass half empty or half full, but we all can agree that we need to fill the glass up. Remember, the goal is to cultivate a growth mindset. Filling the glass up may look like getting a mentor or coach or joining an organization. You need to be deliberate and intentional. Be deliberate with centering yourself among people who are where you want to be in leadership. Be strategic in which healthcare leadership organizations you join. Choose podcasts and conferences that resonate with your goals.

For instance, John C. Maxwell and the *Harvard Business Review* have great leadership content in podcast format. I spend quite a bit of time in the car transporting the kids to and from school and their various activities, and I find that listening to podcasts gives me tools and offers new perspectives on leadership and my interactions with my colleagues. The American College of Healthcare Executives (ACHE) has an annual national conference with timely content and an amazing network. You will find that your leadership gaps will slowly begin to narrow. Colleagues will be refreshed with the enlightened information you are bringing to the boardroom. What level of investment are you willing to make?

I had a mentor, joined the healthcare leadership organization, signed up for conferences, and asked for feedback. I became empowered with resources. Resources are your bridge to closing knowledge gaps. As clinicians, you've mastered learning complex medical concepts—now apply that same discipline to leadership. The key is to be strategic, choosing resources that align with your goals and fit your lifestyle. Podcasts, for instance, are perfect for busy clinicians; a 20-minute episode during a commute can spark a breakthrough idea.

Here's a tool to guide you: **The Resource Road Map**. List three leadership skills you want to develop, like strategic planning or team motivation. For each, identify one resource—a podcast, book, or conference—that targets that skill. For example, for strategic planning, try the *Harvard Business Review*'s podcast or ACHE's leadership workshops. Commit to engaging with one resource per week and applying one insight to your work. Track your progress in a journal to see how your skills grow.

Let's end with a challenge to tie it all together: **The 30-Day Leadership Action Plan**. For the next 30 days, take one daily action aligned with one of these six steps. Day 1: Visualize your leadership identity. Day 2: Reflect on a strength. Day 3: Process a setback, and so on. Journal your actions and their impact. By day 30, you'll have built momentum, confidence, and a clear path to strategic leadership.

This framework is your road map to becoming the leader you're meant to be. Trust your identity, leverage your strengths, rebound from setbacks, align your economics, build your success circle, and empower yourself with resources. You're not just a clinician—you're a visionary ready to transform healthcare. Step into it now.

CHAPTER 8

Leading Yourself First—Sustaining Your Leadership Journey

In order to get to this level of leadership transformation, there are some things that are crucial. It's important to take some time to reflect on your nonnegotiable priorities. Try to see yourself as a whole person, not just in one dimension. Remember, there's more to you than just work; you have families, hobbies, and other interests that are equally important. You shouldn't feel guilty about being at work or at home. Finding a comfortable juggle between your personal life and work life is not easy, but it is doable. This protects you against burnout.

What areas of your life will you absolutely not compromise? You may cherish weekends with family and friends or prefer remote work. You may thrive in teams or in working mostly alone. Traditionally, clinicians have sacrificed and gotten accustomed to sacrificing many things outside of care for our patients. It's time for you, a high-performing clinician, to give the same time and attention to yourself that you effortlessly give to your patients every day.

This step is about reclaiming your wholeness. As a clinician, you're trained to prioritize patients above all else, often at the expense of your own needs. But leadership demands a different approach—one that honors your personal priorities as fiercely as your professional ones. Without this balance, you risk burnout, resentment, or losing sight of why you chose this path. Defining your non-negotiables—whether it's family time, a weekly yoga class, or quiet moments alone—creates a foundation for sustainable leadership.

Let's look at Dr. Brown, an ER physician who stepped into a leadership role overseeing her hospital's emergency services. She loved the challenge but found herself working late nights, missing her kids' soccer games, and feeling drained. She realized her non-negotiable was being home for family dinners for at least three nights a week. By setting this boundary, she restructured her schedule, delegated administrative tasks, and used remote meetings to protect that time. The result? She was more energized at work, her team respected her clarity, and her family felt valued. Dr. Brown's story shows that prioritizing yourself isn't selfish—it's strategic.

Try this tool to clarify your priorities: **The Non-Negotiable Compass**. List three areas of your life you refuse to compromise—family, health, hobbies, or something else. For each, write one action to protect it, like scheduling a weekly family night or blocking an hour for exercise. Review this list weekly to ensure you're honoring these commitments. This compass keeps you grounded, preventing burnout and fueling your leadership longevity.

You need to be okay with not being buddies with everyone. In many instances, our former colleagues have become our direct reports. They will no longer be as transparent as before, and you will need to learn how to assume your role as boss, both at work and afterwards. A mindset shift allowed me to appreciate prior friendship chapters and embrace new relationships in the next chapters. For example, I shared great nights out on the town with some of my colleagues. I still value them as great people, but there are now new boundaries. We enjoy work events with great conversation, but we steer clear of anything further so I can remain objective in my decision-making and not introduce bias. Due to the rapid growth of my leadership journey, I cultivated new friends, where reciprocity in support was provided. I sought out relationships where there was knowledge and/or experience that I had not yet acquired. I, too, have a lot of perspective and experience, and I was thus open to sharing insight with them, creating a symbiotic bidirectional value-added relationship.

Setting boundaries as a leader is both liberating and challenging. As a clinician, you're used to close camaraderie with colleagues, but leadership requires a shift. You can still be warm and approachable, but objectivity is key. This doesn't mean losing connection—it means redefining it. Building new relationships with peers who share your leadership goals can fill the gap, offering mutual support and fresh perspectives.

Here's a practical tool: **The Boundary Builder**. Identify one relationship that needs new boundaries, like a former colleague now reporting to you. Define one action to maintain professionalism, such as limiting social outings or keeping conversations work-focused. Then, seek one new relationship with a fellow leader—perhaps someone from a conference or professional organization. Schedule a coffee chat to exchange insights. This tool helps you navigate the transition from peer to leader while building a supportive network.

In order for this process to work, you have to get real with yourself and get to the point where you do not care as much about the opinions of others. You have to be absolutely sure that this is the right move for you, even when others are delayed getting on board. Quite frankly, some may never get on board with the belief that you can be an impactful leader. Friends, family, or close colleagues may try to convince you to play it safe, even when many people wish they had the courage to step out and take a strategic risk.

When you surround yourself with people who affirm you, the voices of doubt will soon be diminished, and the affirming voices, including your own, will dominate. Trust that you will attract individuals who will breathe life into your new chapter, new goals, and new mindset. Over time, those naysayer opinions will dissipate. You must be able to remind yourself of the cost of not making a move. This is why we went to such effort in chapter 6 to understand the cost of staying put, so price motivates us now to persevere. Go back to the **Vision Clarity Meditation** exercise in chapter 6 to remind yourself of the *why* in pursuing leadership and the cost of not making a move.

Letting go of others' opinions is a superpower. It frees you to pursue your vision without the weight of external judgment. Naysayers—whether colleagues, friends, or even family—may project their own fears onto you. But their doubts don't define your potential. By surrounding yourself with affirmers, as discussed in chapter 7, you amplify your confidence and drown out the noise.

Consider Dr. Marcus, a family practice physician who faced skepticism when he decided to start his own practice. Colleagues questioned why he'd leave a "comfortable" clinical career. Instead of retreating, he leaned on his success circle—a mentor and a peer from a leadership program—who reminded him of his strategic vision. He revisited his chapter 6 exercise, which clarified his *why*: to improve care delivery processes for better patient outcomes. This clarity propelled him forward, and he was successful in building his own practice, proving the naysayers wrong. Dr. Marcus's story shows that your belief in yourself, backed by the right supporters, is stronger than any doubt.

Try this exercise: **The Opinion Filter**. Write down one doubt you've heard about your leadership journey, like "You're too clinical for this role." Next, counter it with evidence of your potential, such as a successful project or a strength from chapter 7. Share this with a trusted affirmer to reinforce your confidence. This filter helps you tune out negativity and focus on your vision.

Your emotional regulation is key. Expect highs and lows with emotions. We can't stop the emotion, but once we feel it, we can regulate it. Much of the regulation has to do with how well we take care of ourselves. Getting enough exercise and sleep will give us the stamina to not let our emotions run wild.

Emotional regulation is the backbone of resilient leadership. As clinicians, you're used to managing high-stakes emotions in patient care, but leadership brings new triggers—criticism, conflicts, or high-pressure decisions. By prioritizing self-care, you build the stamina to stay steady. Exercise, sleep, meditation, or even a hobby like painting can be your anchor, helping you respond thoughtfully rather than react impulsively.

Here's a tool to strengthen this skill: **The Emotional Reset Routine**. Identify one self-care practice that calms you, such as exercise, journaling, or taking a walk. Commit to doing it daily for ten minutes. When you face an emotional challenge, like a tough meeting, use this routine afterward to process your feelings. Then, ask yourself, "What's one constructive step I can take?" This routine keeps your emotions in check and your leadership on track.

In order to do all of the above, you will need to commit to leading yourself first and ensuring your personal wellness tank keeps getting filled back up. There is a certain vibrational state that is necessary for you to carry out the **Dr. Maia Leadership Framework** as a leader and to sustain the proper headspace. Running on a full tank means that when things don't go well, i.e., a presentation bombs, you don't get what you need for staff, folks try to tear down your character, or when conflicts arise across disciplines, you are able to cope a lot better. About three years into my leadership journey, when a colleague spoke negatively about a decision I had made, I could have easily lashed out. However, due to my constant filling up of my wellness tank, I approached it constructively and maintained respect amongst my peers. I did not react. I took in the information and did not respond right away. I went home and thought it through. I was grateful for my direct report who was brave enough to share with me the negative comments she heard. I was able to think about what could have led to him thinking this way. What was his lens? Was there something I failed to see? What could I have been missing in my logic? Is this someone I see as an ally and wish to be on the same page as we both desire to move the organization forward? I ended up having a conversation with this employee and asked him open-ended questions with the intent of active listening.

This story illustrates the power of a full wellness tank. By staying grounded, I turned a potential conflict into a moment of growth. This approach not only preserved my credibility but also strengthened my team's trust. You can do the same by making self-care a non-negotiable, just like your family time or professional goals.

Try this: **The Wellness Tank Checklist**. Create a weekly checklist with three self-care actions—sleep, exercise, and one personal joy (like reading or cooking). Track your consistency and note how it impacts your emotional resilience. For example, after a week of solid sleep, you might notice you handle criticism better. This checklist ensures your tank stays full, empowering you to lead with clarity and calm.

Be sincere about wanting to see the organization thrive with a positive impact on the delivery of care. Yes, you want an opportunity that will provide more money and a seat at the table for decision-making. However, you need to intrinsically get excited about the ultimate reward of being a healthcare leader: helping patients collectively become healthier and live their best lives. This will lead to credibility and cultivating trust amongst peers, direct reports, and patients.

Your sincerity is your secret weapon. It's what makes your leadership authentic and impactful. When you're driven by a genuine desire to improve healthcare, your decisions carry weight, and your team rallies behind you. This passion, combined with your clinical expertise, sets you apart at the leadership table.

Let's wrap up with a challenge: **The 30-Day Leadership Balance Challenge**. For the next 30 days, commit to one daily action that supports your leadership journey while honoring your whole self. Day 1: Define a non-negotiable priority. Day 2: Set a boundary with a colleague. Day 3: Practice an emotional reset. Track your actions in a journal, noting how they make you feel and their impact on your leadership. By day 30, you'll have built a sustainable rhythm that fuels your transformation from clinician to strategic leader.

Leading yourself first is the key to lasting impact. By honoring your priorities, setting boundaries, tuning out naysayers, regulating emotions, and staying grounded in your purpose, you'll not only survive the leadership journey—you'll thrive in it. You are proof that clinical excellence can transform into strategic excellence. Step into it with confidence and let your leadership light shine.

CHAPTER 9

Crafting Your Leadership Path

Let's take a look at your resume. Time to brush it up. What does your resume need to say to accurately reflect your qualifications and readiness for this new job opportunity? Do you need to update your resume? When we think about structuring your resume, make sure it can grab a reader's attention in 90 seconds or less. Standing out from the other applicants will be helpful for you. It's not just a document; it's your career's blockbuster trailer, the pitch that convinces a hiring manager you're the star they've been searching for. Too many resumes are forgettable, like low-budget sequels no one asked for—generic, cluttered, or stuck in the past. But yours? It's going to be a hit. Your resume will scream, "I'm the one you need." By blending storytelling, strategic positioning, and a dash of boldness, you'll craft a resume that's authentic, targeted, and impossible to ignore.

As a clinician transitioning to a leadership role, your resume is more than a list of credentials—it's a narrative that bridges your clinical excellence to your strategic potential. You've spent years mastering patient care, but now you're stepping into a new arena where your ability to influence systems, lead teams, and drive organizational goals takes center stage. Your resume must tell this story with clarity and impact, showcasing not just what you've done but who you are as a leader.

Let's start with a story to set the stage. Dr. Rachel, an Internal Medicine specialist, wanted to transition into a Chief Medical Officer role. Her resume was a dense list of clinical achievements—board certifications, patient outcomes, and research publications. While impressive, it didn't speak to leadership. After researching the job posting and the hospital's mission, she revamped her resume to highlight her success in leading a quality improvement initiative that reduced readmissions by 15%. She added a bold professional summary: "Clinician-leader with a proven track record of driving systemic change and improving patient outcomes." Within weeks, she landed an interview—and eventually, the role. Dr. Rachel's resume didn't just list her skills; it told a story of strategic impact that resonated with her audience.

First, let's talk about your audience—the director of your career movie. Before you touch a single word on your resume, you need to know who's watching. A hiring manager at a tech startup wants to see agility and innovation; a corporate recruiter might prioritize stability and process mastery. Your job is to make your resume speak their language. Dive into the job posting like it's a script, pulling out the top five skills, experiences, or traits the employer values most. If the role calls for "data-driven decision-making," your resume better showcase numbers that prove you've done it. This isn't about guessing—it's about research. Check the company's website, read their mission statement, and scan posts on social media for industry trends. Create a "Job Opportunity Profile" to guide your rewrite. This is your North Star, ensuring every word aligns with what the employer wants.

To create your Job Opportunity Profile, try this exercise: **The Resume Alignment Matrix**. Take the job description for your target role and list its top five requirements—skills, experiences, or qualities like "team leadership" or "strategic planning." Next, match each requirement to a specific achievement from your career. For example, if the role requires "improving operational efficiency," highlight how you streamlined patient flow in your clinic, reducing wait times by 20%. Write a one-sentence bullet point for each match, using action verbs like "spearheaded" or "optimized" and including measurable results. This matrix ensures your resume is laser-focused on the employer's needs, making you an undeniable fit.

Now, let's audit your current resume. Is it a classic or a flop? Most resumes fail because they're outdated, generic, or stuffed with irrelevant details. Pull out your resume and be ruthless. Are you showing impact with specifics like "improved performance metric x by 20%," or are you stuck in vague territory with "responsible for performance outcomes"? Numbers are your box office proof. Is it concise—one to two pages, easy to scan in six seconds? Hiring managers don't have time for a novel. And does it reflect your latest skills, like that new certification in Python or your mastery of AI tools? If your resume feels like it's stuck in 2020, it's time for a reboot. Even if it's solid, tweaking it to match the new job's requirements is nonnegotiable. Highlight the sections that feel outdated or irrelevant, and mark the skills that need more spotlight based on your Job Opportunity Profile.

For clinicians, this audit is especially critical. Your resume likely emphasizes clinical skills—patient care, diagnostics, procedures—but leadership roles demand evidence of strategic impact. Did you lead a team to improve patient satisfaction scores? Did you implement a protocol that saved costs? These are the stories that make hiring managers take notice. If your resume still reads like you're applying for a staff physician role, it's time to shift the narrative.

Here's a tool to guide your audit: **The Resume Impact Scanner**. Print your resume and highlight every bullet point that includes a measurable result (e.g., "increased patient satisfaction by 10%"). If fewer than half your bullets have numbers, rewrite them to include specific outcomes. Next, circle any clinical tasks that don't relate to leadership, like "performed daily rounds." Replace or reframe these to focus on transferable skills, such as "coordinated multidisciplinary teams to ensure seamless patient care." Finally, ensure your resume is scannable—use clear headings, bullet points, and a clean format. This scanner transforms your resume from a clinical checklist to a leadership showcase.

Let's talk about structure. Start with a **professional summary** at the top—a three-to-four-sentence pitch that captures your unique value as a clinician-leader. For example: "Board-certified physician with ten years of clinical excellence, transitioning to strategic leadership with a proven record of improving patient outcomes by 25% through innovative care models." This sets the tone. Follow with a **skills section** highlighting leadership competencies like "change management," "team building," or "data-driven decision-making." Then, list your **professional experience**, prioritizing leadership-related achievements over routine clinical tasks. Use the STAR method (Situation, Task, Action, Result) to craft compelling bullets. For instance: "Led a cross-departmental initiative to reduce ER wait times by 30%, collaborating with nursing and administrative teams to implement streamlined triage protocols." End with **education, certifications,** and **affiliations**, like your membership in the American College of Healthcare Executives (ACHE).

To make this practical, try **The STAR Story Builder**. Choose three career moments that demonstrate leadership—maybe a project you led, a team you motivated, or a policy you influenced. For each, write a one-sentence bullet using the STAR method. For example: "In response to high readmission rates (Situation), tasked with improving patient outcomes (Task), I developed a discharge planning protocol (Action) that reduced readmissions by 15% in six months (Result)." These stories make your resume a compelling narrative, not just a list.

Consider Dr. James, a cardiologist aiming for a medical director role. His original resume was heavy on clinical procedures but light on leadership. After auditing his resume, he added a professional summary: "Clinician with a passion for systemic change, driving a 20% improvement in cardiac care efficiency through team leadership and process innovation." He replaced generic bullets like "managed patient care" with "spearheaded a multidisciplinary task force to enhance care coordination, saving $100,000 annually." His revamped resume landed him multiple interviews, proving the power of strategic storytelling.

Now, let's address the mindset shift. Crafting your resume isn't just about words on a page—it's about owning your identity as a strategic leader. You're not just a clinician; you're a visionary who can transform healthcare. This confidence must shine through in your resume. Avoid self-doubt phrases like "assisted with" or "participated in." Use bold language like "orchestrated" or "drove." Your resume should reflect the same conviction you bring to patient care, signaling to employers that you're ready to lead.

To reinforce this mindset, try **The Leadership Resume Affirmation**. Before revising your resume, write this affirmation: "I am a clinician-leader whose unique expertise transforms organizations and improves lives." Repeat it daily as you work on your resume. This keeps your focus on your strategic value, not just your clinical past.

Finally, let's tie it all together with a challenge: **The 30-Day Resume Transformation Challenge**. For the next 30 days, dedicate time each day to refining your leadership path through your resume. Day 1: Create your Job Opportunity Profile. Day 5: Audit your resume with the Impact Scanner. Day 10: Write a professional summary. Day 20: Craft three STAR stories. By day 30, you'll have a resume that screams leadership and positions you as the top candidate. Track your progress in a journal, noting how your confidence grows with each step.

Your resume is your ticket to the leadership table. It's not just a document—it's your story of transformation from clinical excellence to strategic excellence. Craft it with intention, align it with your audience, and let it boldly declare: "I am proof." The healthcare world is waiting for your leadership—make sure your resume opens the door.

CHAPTER 10

Making Your Mark—Leading with Impact and Legacy

You've crafted your leadership path, polished your resume, and embraced the mindset shift from clinician to strategic thinker. Now, it's time to take the leap and make your mark. This chapter isn't about waiting for the perfect moment or hoping someone hands you the keys to leadership—it's about stepping boldly into your role, building influence, and creating a legacy that transforms healthcare. As a clinician-leader, your impact isn't measured by the patients you treat in a day but by the systems you improve, the teams you inspire, and the lasting change you leave behind. This is your moment to prove you are ready to lead, not just today, but for the long haul.

The final step in our **Dr. Maia Leadership Framework** is about action—deliberate, courageous, and strategic action. You've built the foundation: You trust your identity (chapter 7), know your strengths, rebound from setbacks, align your economics, value your success circle, and empower yourself with resources. You've let go of needing everyone's approval and prioritized your wellness (chapter 8). You've crafted a resume that screams leadership (chapter 9). Now, it's time to put it all into motion. Leadership isn't a destination; it's a journey of consistent, intentional steps that ripple outward, creating impact far beyond the exam room.

STEP 1: TAKE BOLD ACTION

The first step to making your mark is to act. Bold action doesn't mean reckless leaps—it means taking calculated steps toward your vision, even when fear whispers to hold back. As a clinician, you're used to making quick, high-stakes decisions in patient care. Now, apply that decisiveness to leadership. Whether it's proposing a new protocol, volunteering for a committee, or applying for a leadership role, the time to act is now.

Here's a tool to get you moving: **The Bold Action Blueprint**. Identify one leadership goal, like leading a quality improvement project or securing a medical director role. Break it into three actionable steps you can take within the next 30 days. Consider this example:

1. Schedule a meeting with a decision-maker to pitch your idea.
2. Prepare a one-page proposal with data and outcomes.
3. Follow up with a thank-you email and next steps. Write these steps in a journal and commit to completing them.

Each action builds momentum, proving to yourself and others that you're a leader in motion.

STEP 2: BUILD INFLUENCE THROUGH RELATIONSHIPS

Leadership isn't about titles—it's about influence. As a clinician-leader, your ability to inspire, persuade, and collaborate sets you apart. This means building relationships with stakeholders across the organization—executives, colleagues, and staff. Your clinical background gives you a unique edge: You understand the front lines of care, which makes your voice powerful. But influence requires intentionality.

Consider Dr. Michael, an anesthesiologist who wanted to improve efficiency. He noticed tensions between specialists and administrative staff over scheduling conflicts. Instead of pushing his own agenda, he built relationships by listening to both sides, hosting informal lunches to gather insights, and proposing a collaborative solution that cut scheduling delays by 25%. His influence grew because he showed he valued everyone's perspective. Today, he's a trusted advisor to his hospital's C-suite, all because he invested in relationships.

Try this exercise: **The Influence Map**. List five key stakeholders in your organization—perhaps a department head, a nurse manager, or a board member. For each, write one way you can build a connection, like inviting them to coffee or acknowledging their work in a meeting. Over the next two weeks, take one action per stakeholder. Reflect on how these connections strengthen your influence. This map turns relationships into a powerful tool for leadership impact.

STEP 3: COMMUNICATE WITH IMPACT

Your voice is your superpower. As a clinician, you've honed your ability to communicate with patients and families. Now, translate that clarity and empathy into leadership communication. Whether you're presenting a proposal, leading a meeting, or advocating for change, your ability to articulate your vision with confidence and authenticity will set you apart.

Here's a tool to sharpen your communication: **The Impactful Message Framework**. Before any high-stakes conversation or presentation, answer three questions:

1. What's my core message? (e.g., "This initiative will improve patient outcomes by 15%.")
2. Why does it matter to my audience? (e.g., "It aligns with our mission to enhance care quality.")
3. What action do I want them to take? (e.g., "Approve funding for this pilot.")

Write a concise pitch based on these answers and practice it aloud. This framework ensures your message is clear, compelling, and action-oriented.

Dr. Sofia, a Nurse Practitioner, used this approach to secure funding for a telemedicine program. She crafted a pitch that tied her data-driven proposal to the hospital's patient-centered mission, ending with a clear call to action. Her presentation won over the board, and her program became a model for other hospitals. Your voice can do the same—use it to inspire and drive change.

STEP 4: MEASURE AND CELEBRATE YOUR IMPACT

Leadership isn't just about action—it's about results. As a clinician-leader, you're uniquely positioned to measure impact through metrics like patient outcomes, team performance, or cost savings. Tracking your results not only validates your work but also builds your credibility. Equally important is celebrating your wins, no matter how small. This fuels your motivation and inspires others to follow your lead.

Try this tool: **The Impact Tracker**. Choose one leadership project or goal, like improving patient flow or mentoring a team. Define one measurable outcome, such as "reduce wait times by 10%" or "increase team engagement scores by 5%." Track your progress weekly in a journal, noting milestones and challenges. When you hit a milestone, celebrate—share the win with your team, treat yourself to a coffee, or reflect on your growth. This tracker keeps you focused and energized.

Dr. Raj, an emergency physician, used this approach when leading a triage overhaul. He tracked wait time reductions weekly, sharing updates with his team. When they hit a 15% improvement, he celebrated with a team lunch, boosting morale and reinforcing their shared success. Celebrating impact isn't just feel-good—it's a leadership strategy that builds momentum.

STEP 5: BUILD YOUR LEGACY

Leadership is about more than immediate results—it's about the legacy you leave. As a clinician-leader, your legacy is the lasting change you create in healthcare, whether it's better patient care, empowered teams, or innovative systems. Think beyond your current role: What mark do you want to leave on your organization, community, or the broader field of healthcare?

Try this exercise: **The Legacy Vision Statement**. Write a one-paragraph vision of the legacy you want to leave in five years. For example: "I want to be known as a leader who transformed patient access by implementing equitable care models and mentoring the next generation of clinician-leaders." Revisit this statement monthly, asking, "What's one action I took this month toward this legacy?" This keeps your focus on long-term impact.

STEP 6: STAY COMMITTED TO GROWTH

The leadership journey doesn't end—it evolves. To sustain your impact, commit to continuous growth. This means seeking feedback, staying curious, and adapting to the ever-changing healthcare landscape. Your clinical training taught you to stay current with medical advances; now, apply that same discipline to leadership. Join organizations like ACHE, listen to leadership podcasts, or invest in coaching to keep sharpening your skills.

In my **Dr. Maia Leadership Framework** program, I guide clients to create a growth plan tailored to their leadership goals. For example, one client, Dr. Lee, committed to attending one leadership webinar monthly and seeking feedback after every major presentation. Within a year, he went from feeling like an outsider in boardroom discussions to leading them with confidence. Your growth is your fuel—keep investing in it.

Here's a tool to stay on track: **The Growth Commitment Plan**. List ways you'll invest in your leadership growth over the next six months—perhaps joining a professional organization, reading a leadership book, or finding a mentor. Schedule one action per month and track your progress. For instance, if you join ACHE, attend their next webinar and apply one insight to your work. This plan ensures you're always evolving as a leader.

THE 30-DAY LEADERSHIP IMPACT CHALLENGE

Let's tie it all together with a challenge to make your mark: **The 30-Day Leadership Impact Challenge**. For the next 30 days, take one daily action aligned with these steps. Day 1: Create your Bold Action Blueprint. Day 5: Build one relationship from your Influence Map. Day 10: Practice your Impactful Message Framework. Day 15: Track a milestone with your Impact Tracker. Day 20: Write your Legacy Vision Statement. Day 25: Schedule a growth action from your Growth Commitment Plan. Journal each action and its impact on your confidence and influence. By day 30, you'll see tangible proof of your leadership in action.

You are ready to make your mark. Your clinical expertise, combined with your strategic mindset, positions you to transform healthcare in ways others can't. Don't wait for permission or perfection—take bold action, build influence, communicate with impact, measure your results, create your legacy, and commit to growth. You are not just a clinician—you are a leader, a change maker, and a legacy builder. The healthcare world needs your voice, and the time to act is now. Step into your power and prove you are the leader you were meant to be.

CONCLUSION

Your Time to Thrive

In order to THRIVE as a clinician-leader, you need to decide that now is the time to shift from individualized patient care excellence toward strategic organizational excellence, clear vision, and alignment with personal strengths and non-negotiables. Trust your Leadership Identity—envision where you want to be, affirm yourself, and respond to naysayers. It will be scary, and I am here to help you. I want to share with you the land mines that were not shared with me. I want to help you figure out the road map that makes sense for you to achieve your dreams. Let's set achievable goals and milestones so that you can expedite your transformation. It doesn't have to be scary, and you do not have to be alone. Book a call with me at www.DrMaia.coach so we can chat more about where you are on your journey. Look for tools, leadership tips, and conversations on my website, www.DrMaia.coach.

This journey you've embarked on through these pages is about more than a career pivot—it's about stepping into the fullness of who you are meant to be. You are a clinician, yes, but you are also a visionary, a change maker, and a leader poised to transform healthcare. The mindset shift from practitioner to strategic thinker (chapter 4) is your key to unlocking a life of impact, fulfillment, and legacy. You've learned to trust your identity (chapter 1), leverage your unique strengths (chapter 2 and chapter 7), reframe hurdles as opportunities (chapter 3) rebound from setbacks, align your economics, build a success circle, and empower yourself with resources (chapter 7). You've embraced boundaries, tuned out doubt (chapter 5) and prioritized your wellness (chapter 8). You've crafted a resume that screams leadership (chapter 9) and taken bold action to make your mark (chapter 6). Now, it's time to bring it all together and launch into your leadership legacy (chapter 10).

Let me share a story to anchor this moment. Dr. Karey, an internist with a passion for patient advocacy, felt trapped in her clinical role. She yearned to influence hospital policy. She doubted her readiness for leadership, fearing her lack of experience would hold her back. But after working through my **Dr. Maia Leadership Coaching** program, she clarified her vision: to lead a policy that improved access to mental health services. She started by affirming her strengths—empathy and strategic problem-solving—and she built a network of allies, including a mentor who guided her through boardroom dynamics. When she pitched her initiatives, the hospital board listened. Today, she's a director of patient services, shaping policies that touch thousands of lives. Dr. Karey's transformation began with a decision: to stop waiting and to start leading. That same decision is yours to make now.

This is your moment to decide that you are ready to thrive—not tomorrow, not after another degree, but right now. The healthcare system needs your voice, your perspective, and your unique ability to bridge clinical excellence with strategic vision. You don't need to have all the answers; you need the courage to take the first step, the resilience to keep going, and the wisdom to seek support. That's why I'm here—to walk alongside you, to help you navigate the land mines I stumbled over, and to guide you toward a road map that's as unique as you are.

Let's make this personal. Pause for a moment and imagine yourself one year from now. Where are you? Perhaps you're leading a department, presenting a game-changing initiative, or mentoring a team of clinicians. Picture the confidence in your walk, the clarity in your voice, the impact of your decisions. Now, ask yourself: What's the cost of not starting today? In chapter 6, you reflected on your *why* and the risks of staying put. Revisit that exercise now. The price of inaction—missed opportunities, unfulfilled potential, a healthcare system that lacks your voice—is too high. You deserve a life where your work aligns with your strengths, honors your non-negotiables, and creates a legacy you're proud of.

Here's a tool to solidify your commitment: **The Leadership Launch Plan**. Take a piece of paper and write down three specific actions you'll take within the next 30 days to launch your leadership journey. These could be booking a call with me at www.DrMaia.coach, joining a leadership organization like ACHE, or proposing a small initiative at work. For each action, set a deadline and one person you'll share it with for accountability—perhaps a mentor or peer from your success circle (chapter 7). This plan transforms your decision into tangible steps, ensuring you don't just dream of leadership—you live it.

Now, let's address the fear. Yes, it's scary to step into uncharted territory. I remember my first leadership role, feeling like all eyes were on me, waiting for me to prove myself. The naysayers were loud—colleagues who doubted a clinician could lead, peers who urged me to "play it safe." But I learned to respond, not react. I surrounded myself with affirmers, as we discussed in (chapter 8), who drowned out the noise with encouragement and belief. You can do the same. When doubt creeps in, revisit your strengths (chapter 7), affirm your vision, and lean on your success circle. You are not alone, and you are more ready than you know.

To make this mindset shift stick, try this exercise: **The Affirmation Anchor**. Write down this affirmation: "I am a clinician-leader, uniquely equipped to transform healthcare with my vision and expertise." Say it aloud every morning for the next week, standing tall with your shoulders back. Notice how it shifts your energy, grounding you in your leadership identity. Share this affirmation with a trusted colleague or friend, asking them to remind you of it when you waver. This anchor keeps you centered, especially on tough days.

THE LEADERSHIP PRESCRIPTION WORKBOOK

Leadership is built through application. Scan here for the strategic workbook.

WHAT TO DO NEXT

Remember that your first step is to decide that the time is right now to launch into leadership. You have waited long enough, and now is the time to have the life you want. Tap into the leader that is already inside of you. Affirm yourself with a positive mindset. Dig deep to understand your strengths and where you excel. This will ensure you pursue opportunities that will grant you the most success and fulfillment. Cultivate an environment of other leaders in close proximity to you and acquire resources that will aid you in your leadership pursuit.

I invite you to go to my website at www.DrMaia.coach. Book a call with me at www.DrMaia.coach/book-call-7839-4813. Let's review your results from your 30-Day challenges. It would be my pleasure to coach you.

ABOUT THE AUTHOR

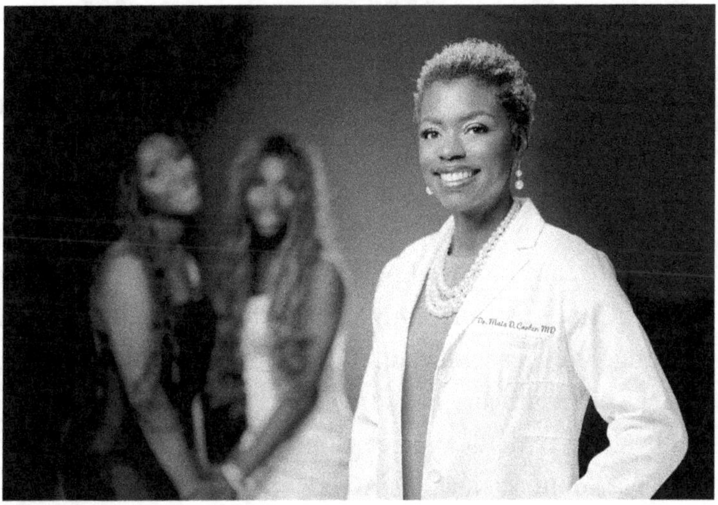

Dr. Maia Carter is a board-certified internal medicine physician and a coach to clinicians and healthcare leaders. She has worked in the federal sector for over 16 years and has been a physician leader holding various leadership roles for over 10 years. She serves as an outpatient primary care physician and is currently a national director driving implementation and expansion of virtual tools for primary care teams. Renowned for her transparency, relatability, and visionary approach to leadership, whether she is leading her community, guiding groups of clinicians, or guesting on a podcast, Dr. Carter's insights resonate deeply with her audience. She specializes in helping frontline clinicians become influential leaders without burning out or losing their clinical edge. With over a decade of experience leading healthcare teams, developing physician executives, and mentoring early-career physicians, Dr. Carter brings warmth, clarity, and strategic thinking to every stage she graces. She has spoken for a variety of groups and professional associations, such as the Southern Nevada Health District (SNHD), American College of Healthcare Executives (ACHE), and the American College of Physicians (ACP). She holds an MD and MPH from The George Washington University and completed her BS in Physiology from Michigan State University. She completed a preventive cardiology fellowship at Saint Luke's Hospital in Kansas City, Missouri, immediately following her medical training. She has achieved fellow status with the American College of Healthcare Executives and the American College of Physicians. Medical career highlights include serving as 2024 president of Nevada's ACHE chapter and service chair of the Red Shoe Society, a philanthropic organization that supports Ronald McDonald House Charities (RMHC). Her groundbreaking leadership coaching program, Dr. Maia Leadership Framework, Dr. Maia Enterprises, LLC, offers a personalized approach to transform overwhelmed providers into strategic powerhouses who are equipped to lead with vision, authenticity, and purpose.

But Dr. Maia's story is more than her credentials; it's a testament to the power of transformation. Once a frontline clinician navigating the relentless demands of patient care, she faced the same doubts and burnout that many of you feel. She wondered if leadership was possible without sacrificing her passion for medicine or her personal life. That pivotal moment came when she decided to shift her mindset from practitioner to strategic thinker, a journey that led her to redefine success not by patients seen but by systems transformed and lives uplifted. This book, *The Leadership Prescription*, is born from that journey. It's her proof that clinicians can become visionary leaders who shape healthcare's future while staying true to their calling.

Dr. Maia's path wasn't always smooth. Early in her leadership journey, she stumbled, feeling isolated in boardrooms where her clinical perspective seemed out of place. But she leaned into her strengths—empathy, resilience, and a knack for connecting with people, and she sought mentors and coaches who showed her how to bridge clinical and strategic worlds. Those lessons became the foundation of her **Dr. Maia Leadership Coaching** program, where she coaches clinicians to overcome fear, align with their purpose, and step boldly into roles like Chief Medical Officer, Medical Director, or Policy Influencer. Her clients don't just survive leadership; they thrive, creating legacies that ripple through their organizations and communities.

What sets Dr. Maia apart is her heart. Whether she's speaking to a packed auditorium at an ACHE conference or coaching a single clinician over Zoom, she brings warmth, authenticity, and a relentless belief in your potential. She's walked the path you're on, faced the naysayers, and emerged stronger, proving that leadership isn't about perfection—it's about courage and impact. Her work supporting families through the Red Shoe

Society and Ronald McDonald House Charities reflects her commitment to community, while her roles in ACHE showcase her influence in shaping healthcare leadership nationwide.

Dr. Maia's mission is clear: to empower you, the aspiring clinician-leader, with the **Dr. Maia Leadership Framework**. Through *The Leadership Prescription*, she shares the road map she wished she'd had, packed with tools, stories, and strategies to navigate the leadership leap. But this book is just the beginning. She invites you to join her community at www.DrMaia.coach, where you can book a call to map out your leadership journey and receive practical tips and inspiring conversations. Her **Dr. Maia Leadership Framework** offers personalized coaching to transform your vision into reality, ensuring you lead with confidence, avoid burnout, and make a lasting impact.

Dr. Maia Carter is more than a physician, coach, or speaker—she's proof that your clinical expertise can ignite strategic excellence. She's here to guide you past the land mines, cheer your wins, and help you build a life of purpose and influence. Take the first step today: Visit www.DrMaia.coach, connect with her, and make your leadership dreams unstoppable. Dr. Maia is ready to help you shine.

www.ingramcontent.com/pod-product-compliance
Lightning Source LLC
LaVergne TN
LVHW022100200926
848481LV00003B/1001
* 9 7 9 8 9 9 4 8 4 4 5 0 2 *